Praise for
MOON TIME

This book is a wonderful journey of discovery. Lucy not only guides us through the wisdom inherent in our wombs, our cycles and our hearts, but also encourages us to share, express, celebrate and enjoy what it means to be female!
A beautiful and inspiring book full of practical information and ideas.
Miranda Gray, author *Red Moon* and *The Optimized Woman*

Lucy, your book, Moon Time, is monumental. I cannot tell you how long I have thought of the very things you are putting forward, and to see this in print is thrilling.
Moon Time is a well needed resource book covering a wide range of important ways to respect our blood cycles wisely. Holding our cycles, bodies, and stages in life with the highest regard breaks the spell of centuries of oppression where our blood has been considered a dirty curse. The wisdom in Moon Time sets a new course where we glimpse a future culture reshaped by honoring our womanhood journeys one woman at a time.
Cozy up, get yourself a cup of tea and come home as a daughter of the Red River flowing.
ALisa Starkweather,
founder of Red Tent Temple Movement.
Co-author *The Red Tent Movement: A Historical Perspective* and
Women, Spirituality and Transformative Leadership

Lucy Pearce weaves a moon-web that draws in the many other women who have written on the subject of menstrual cycles and places herself as one, amongst others. Her open and accessible book offers practical, often humorous ideas and encouragement about how we can tune into our own cycles and 'dance' with them in the most creative and healthy way.

She is one of the special whisperers, who helps us to remember our own power and sacredness as played out in our cycles. Through her writing she initiates a dialogue with her readers. Her writing empowers her readers to have a voice to respond. This is a remarkable gift to us.

**Tracy Evans, PhD researcher, women's rites of passage,
University of Aberystwyth**

Moon Time *is a beautifully written resource for deepening your connection with your cycle. Full of personal heartfelt suggestions, simple rituals and practical ways to support women in understanding the influence their hormones have on them each month.*
This book could change your life!

**Rachael Hertogs, compiling editor of *Thirteen Moons*
and author *Menarche: A Journey to Womanhood***

MOON TIME

Other books by the same author

Burning Woman

Full Circle Health: integrated health charting for women

Moon Time: harness the ever-changing energy of your menstrual cycle

The Rainbow Way: cultivating creativity in the midst of motherhood

Moods of Motherhood: the inner journey of mothering

Burning Woman: an initiation to feminine power

Anthology Contributor

Earth Pathways Diary 2011–16

Musing on Mothering mothersmilkbooks.com (2012)

Tiny Buddha's Guide to Loving Yourself Hay House (2013)

Roots: Where Food Comes From and Where It Takes Us: A Blogher Anthology (2013)

If Women Rose Rooted, Sharon Blackie (2016)

She Rises: Vol. 2 Mago Books (2016)

MOON TIME

Harness the ever-changing
energy of your menstrual cycle

Lucy H. Pearce

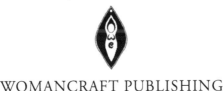

WOMANCRAFT PUBLISHING

Cover art by Elena Ray
Typeset and design by Lucent Word
www.lucentword.com

Extended quotations used with the express permission of their authors.

The advice contained in this book is provided as information only, not formal medical or contraceptive guidance. It is recommended that you seek further professional advice.

Second edition published by Womancraft Publishing, 2015
www.womancraftpublishing.com

ISBN: 978-1910559-062 (paperback)
ISBN: 978-1910559-079 (ebook)

For my mother:
I am me,
Because you were you.

ACKNOWLEDGEMENTS

Welcome to the second edition of *Moon Time*, just over three years after its initial publication.

I am honoured and delighted that this little book, my first, which was initially written as a small personal project, has been received with so much love and gratitude by women around the world.

It was this book that made me an author... and publisher. That women who did not know me trusted me enough to buy it was miraculous to me. That it has become the consistently #1 bestselling book on menstruation on Amazon.com is beyond my wildest dreams.

It has brought me into contact with the leading ladies in the world of women's health and for that I am profoundly grateful. It has brought me speaking and teaching engagements. And with each I have built my understanding of menstruation, red tents and emergent women's culture. These are exciting times we are living in, and I am so honoured to have become part of this movement.

Each week I am moved to receive emails from readers around the world expressing gratitude for this little book. 'Life changing' is an expression I hear quite regularly, and one I am always humbled by.

I wish to thank all those who have supported my writing and my life as they have unfolded:

My mother, Francesca, for giving me life, and making me who I am.

My father, Stephen, for providing the template for making a

living from honouring your creativity. And for creating and sharing the tea house where this book was first written.

My grandmothers, Lucy and Suzanne, who shaped me more than they could possibly know, and whose physical presence I miss deeply, but whose spirits are always by my side.

My step-mother, Lauren: part mother, part sister, part friend, but as far from wicked as it's possible to get!

My sister Mirin, for blossoming into the young woman I always wished I had been, right in front of my eyes.

My best school friend, Emma, with whom I shared the news of my first bleeding and the joy of my first birth, as well as many other secrets along the way.

My women's group: Amy, Meadhbh, Delphine, Louise, Mary, Sharon, Leigh and Loo for holding the container of our collective womb within which we have all grown.

My soul sisters: Tracy, Mary, Leigh, Laura and Paula. For seeing me as I am—and celebrating that with me.

The many, many open-hearted, shining souled women and men I have met on this journey of writing and teaching—whose insights, appreciation, and experiences have helped me to grow.

My treasured readers at Dreaming Aloud and *Juno* and tribe of inspirational women on Facebook who helped me to develop the cover, subtitle and resources section for this second edition.

ALisa, Miranda, Lorraine, Rachael, Nicholas, Isadora, Shawn, Zoë and Dawn for their beautiful work and generous, open-hearted permission to reproduce it in this book. Your blessings for my work have touched my soul.

My husband, Patrick, for his technical prowess—everything I don't know how to do, he does—we make a good team! For supporting my women's work and creativity, for being open to sharing working and childcare, for keeping me sane and helping me to laugh over the years, I am incredibly grateful. You truly are my soft place to fall.

And finally to our three children: Timmy, Merrily and Aisling, for their patience with me when the Crazy Woman roams, my distractedness when a creative project is gestating, as well as for their love and the fun that we share. I am so glad to be your mother.

CONTENTS

INTRODUCTION

Welcome, dearest woman.

I am so glad you're here. Are you ready for an adventure? The location isn't a far-off land, but somewhere much closer to home: your beautiful body. And your compass is your menstrual cycle.

Despite having inhabited them our whole lives, our bodies can often feel very foreign to us. We can feel out of control, at the mercy of our own hormones, never knowing whether we'll be full of energy or curling up in a ball, exhausted and aching.

Our female bodies are quixotic—our energy levels, moods and physical health constantly changing. It can feel disorientating and frustrating. But what's worse is there seems to be little support or acknowledgement of this reality. We're supposed to just ignore it all and carry on regardless.

It is my guess that no one ever initiated you into the path of womanhood. Instead, just like me, you were left to find out by yourself. Little by little you pieced a working understanding of your body and soul together. But still you have gaps.

You yearn for a greater knowledge of your woman's body, a comprehensive understanding of who you are, why you are that way.

Perhaps you have searched long and hard, seeking advice from your mother, sister, aunts and friends, tired of suffering and struggling alone. You may have visited doctors, healers or therapists, but still you feel at sea and your woman's body is a mystery to you.

Or maybe you have never given your cycles a second thought. . . until now.

Perhaps you are seeking. . .

- ○ deeper harmony with yourself and your cycle

- ○ greater self-knowledge and self-acceptance

- ○ to better understand your fertility and make new contraceptive choices

- ○ to improve your experience of 'that time of the month'

- ○ a way to balance your hectic life and your body's needs

- ○ to heal your womb

- ○ to harness your ever-changing energy to improve your creativity, working life or relationships

- ○ positive language to describe your body and its functions

- ○ a practical guide to creating a red tent or moon lodge

- ○ natural ways of dealing with PMS

- ○ ideas for celebrating the next part of womanhood that you, or your daughter, are entering

- ○ a greater physical connection to nature's cycles, seasons and the moon

This book will help you with all these and more.

Through knowledge we gain power over our lives.

With options we have possibility.

With acceptance we find a new freedom.

Why our cycles matter

We start bleeding earlier today than ever before, with girls' first periods occurring at 12.8 years old now, compared with 14.5 years at the beginning of the last century. Coupled with lower breastfeeding rates, better nutrition and fewer pregnancies, women now menstruate more in their adult lives than at any time in our history.

Menstruation matters.

From the age of 12 to 51, unless you are pregnant or on the pill, every single day of your life as a woman is situated somewhere on the menstrual cycle. Whether ovulating or bleeding, struggling with PMS or conception, our bodies, our energy levels, our sense of self, even our abilities are constantly shifting each and every day.

And yet nobody talks about it.

Everyone just ignores it. Women are expected to be the same, day in, day out. Despite the fact that our bodies are cycling through the various parts of the menstrual cycle.

Just keep calm and carry on.

As girls we may have been taught to look out for our first blood. And told what to use to absorb it. But after that: silence. Hide it, ignore it. . . and make sure no one notices.

And so we think we must be a little crazy as we experience these massive fluctuations every month. Unless we're lucky enough to have a close girlfriend who shares her inner world with us. But many of us don't. And so we are alone in our bodies.

Take what works. . . and leave the rest

This book walks on tender ground. Each woman comes to it with her own sensitivities and unique experiences, her own pains and pre-conceptions. Not everything here might be resonant with you. Perhaps you are just beginning the journey of self-acceptance, just starting to learn about your body's cycles. Or perhaps you have been studying them for years and are seeking resources to help you dig deeper into yourself, to empower you to share your journey and wisdom with other women in your community.

Whatever your starting point, whatever your background, I honour you, and want this book to be deeply accessible and acceptable to you.

When we come across new ideas which challenge the way we have learned to see the world and ourselves we can be triggered. We can feel judgement, shame, anger. . . The new information is like a red flag: either *it* must be wrong. . . or *we* must be wrong. Most of us don't like to be wrong. It makes us feel threatened and unsafe.

I want you to feel safe, my love. And I want you to learn and grow too. That's why you picked up this book.

So if I suggest something which doesn't sit well with you, I invite you to examine it:

- o Is it uncomfortable to you simply because it is a new idea?

- o Is it something you have been taught to reject or disapprove of?

- o Is it something which you feel others might judge you on, or ridicule?

- o Is it something you have tried and know you don't like?

- o Or are we coming from different assumptions or understandings?

To thine own self be true

As you work through this book, be true to yourself. I cannot lead you towards self-knowledge. Only you can do that. I can offer candles and matches. But you must light them.

Let this book sow the seeds—and then explore the ideas further: Google them, ask friends and practitioners, question them, try them out in your own life and see if the ideas and activities 'grow corn' for you. Do they work? Do they heal you? Do they help you feel more connected to yourself, and to the people in your life? If so, then they are good and right for you.

If I suggest something that you hate then rather than just reacting against it, ask yourself: what about it feels wrong for me? What would be a more acceptable, exciting alternative for me? And then go make it happen. Go create your own uniquely wonderful path to healing and wholeness.

It is my deepest wish to help you to celebrate you, your body and help you to reconnect with your female rhythms. This book offers you hundreds of different ways in. All it takes is one to start you on your own path, or unblock the way.

Start small

With much of this women's work, because it goes against the grain of what we have been taught in our culture, many of us find that it is easier to start small and private, whilst we are still learning and growing. There is less vulnerability, less opportunity to shame ourselves or be shamed by others in our early experiments. Others need the support and encouragement of a group of like-minded women as they explore these new terrains. Again, do what works for you.

Take your time.

Be gentle with yourself,

and all those that you meet on the path.

Remember that you are not alone. All around the world, over two billion women are travelling this path: silent sisters of the moon. Through this book you will learn how to kindle your own wisdom flame, and share it together with your daughters and sisters and communities. You will find ways to celebrate and support each other, break our silence about what it means to live in a woman's body in this world.

So here we are, at the beginning of our journey together, to explore the mystery of being a woman.

My journey

I always find it helps on a journey to know a little about my companion and where she has come from, so that we can travel in trust and ease together.

I am the mother of three children (currently aged nine, seven and five). I have been working in women's work for the past nine years, running women's circles, mother blessing ceremonies and holistic birth preparation classes. I helped to set up a women's group and red tent here in my area. I have written on women's issues (natural pregnancy, birth, motherhood, moon time, creativity and health) for nearly a decade in my career as a freelance writer, author of four books, blogger and contributing editor at *Juno* magazine.

Whilst many of my credentials are quite alternative, and many chalk me down as 'New Age', I am not, if truth be told, that comfortable with anything too 'out there'. For me everything must be firmly grounded and integrated. The thrust of my work is, and always has been, to bring what works from alternative circles back into the mainstream, to integrate wisdom with science and to make it accessible to all.

I have been on this journey of menstrual exploration for 15 years now.

My initiation was at 20, struggling with being on the pill and hating it. I came across the book *Women's Bodies, Women's Wisdom* which set me on a path of curiosity and discovery about my own female body. That book has changed my life many times over.

That was the beginning. But my embodied transition to awareness really happened as a result of gestating, birthing and breastfeeding three children. There is nothing like being caught in the endless cycle of procreation for seven years to put you in touch with your body and how it works!

Coming back to my periods after prolonged breaks each time gave me a chance to be more reflective and aware of them rather than simply reacting to them. I began to see how my body and its fertility impacted my creative and sexual energies, through pregnancy, post-partum and my cycles. I began to connect the dots in my personal experience—dots that my culture had never even told me were there.

I became aware from first-hand experience of the power of my womb to create, hold and give birth to life. I understood its function. The point of periods was no longer abstract, and my sexuality was not just for fun, or limited by fear of pregnancy. As I witnessed this first in myself, and then in the women I worked alongside, I developed an ever greater sense of gratitude and compassion for myself and all women. As well as a sadness that this wisdom is not acknowledged or supported in our culture.

I have many different moods to my physical and emotional life, and so I have learnt to celebrate them rather than ignore them. To co-create with them rather than resist them. This truly has been a wonderful journey, which has impacted my work, life and relationships in so many ways.

And I am still learning. Still uncovering new depth and insight—through my lived experience and in books. I am an apprentice to my body. Some days more successful than others!

Often I get impatient and push and force myself. I ignore what I know and everyone suffers—me, my husband and kids. I feel like a slow learner. But then I look around me and almost all the women I know of my age, and older, are in this place of learning. And I remind myself to be gentle and compassionate with myself, not to shame myself. Because we are not initiated into what it means to become a woman.

What does it mean to be a woman?

Despite coming from a loving home, I was sensitive to a lot of messages to do with being a woman that went unspoken (and unchallenged) in the world at large. These were the things I learned subconsciously from our culture about being a woman.

(Why not tick off those which are true for you too!)

○ To be a woman is *to be less than*. That's why we aren't represented in anywhere near equal numbers anywhere—from history books, to the halls of government, to TV comedy shows. And why lots of the insults you can call someone are female too.

○ Women's bodies are unreliable.

○ Women have a lot to be ashamed about. Body hair, imperfect bodies, aging. . . If you're not perfect hide it away, don't talk about it, be silent and for goodness' sake be discrete.

○ If you really experience serious pain (and are not just imagining it or attention-seeking) then go to a doctor to help you silence your symptoms.

○ Wombs cause pain, that's what they do, they're faulty objects to be tolerated or removed. Stop moaning and get on with it.

○ Women bleed. Menstruation is embarrassing, dirty, taboo, shameful and unclean.

○ The menstrual cycle is an irrelevant inconvenience and certainly not of any relevance or importance to us or our world.

○ Women are weak, unreliable and over-emotional especially when they are 'on the rag'. This is a valid topic for multiple smutty jokes.

○ It is preferable to avoid menstruation. It is a problem which most women would like to be rid of.

○ Periods prevent us from being fully functional or rational, and so unable to play roles of importance in a man's world.

○ Don't get pregnant! (Until you're 30).

○ Or why can't you get pregnant? (If you're over 30).

○ Mothering is not an important or valued role.

○○○

Throughout the book you will find '**AND YOU?**' sections which invite you to reflect and respond, to apply what you have read to yourself. Perhaps you would like to note answers to the questions briefly in your journal. Perhaps some call you to a longer, more detailed response. Or maybe you just want to answer them in your head as you read. As with the rest of this book, do what works for you!

AND YOU?

What does it mean to you to be a woman?

What were you taught... and what have you learnt through experience?

Which of these lessons are true for you?

Are there any more lessons that you would add?

Which of these do you still believe or live by?

Which have you rejected?

How do you feel about your cycles at the moment?

How has this evolved over the years?

There is little understanding and allowance for the realities of being a cycling woman—let alone celebration.

But that changes here!

Take my hand. . . Let us begin!

OUR CYCLES:
A BIOLOGICAL UNDERSTANDING

How much did you learn about your menstrual cycle in school? Most of us learned about our female biology in science classes, from a detached perspective—full of big scientific words and abstract diagrams—which often felt like it had little to do with us.

We are not taught in school about the experiential aspects of our cycles, or the spiritual and intuitive gifts of menstruation. Before we dive deeper into the wisdom of our cycles, we first need to make sure that we're all on the same page about what actually happens to our bodies during the menstrual cycle. Understanding the biology and physiology of our cycles is the first key to acceptance and living in balance with all the processes that go on unseen within us.

Each month our bodies go through a series of changes, many of which we may be unconscious of. These include: shifts in levels of hormones, vitamins and minerals, vaginal temperature and secretions, the structure of the womb lining and cervix, body weight, water retention, heart rate, breast size and texture, attention span, pain threshold. . .

The changes are biological. Measurable. They are most definitely not 'all in your head' as many would have us believe. This is why it is so crucial to honour these changes by adapting our lives to them as much as possible.

We cannot just will these changes not to happen as they are an integral part of our fertility.

Menstruation

O **Day one** is the first day of bleeding. The bleeding occurs when the nutrient-rich womb lining disintegrates and is shed because no egg has been implanted.

O This usually lasts four to six days getting lighter in the final couple of days.

O Only an egg-cup full of blood is lost, but it looks like a lot more!

O If you are taking the pill, the bleeding that you experience is not a menstrual period but simply a withdrawal bleed from the artificially induced state of quasi-pregnancy that the hormones create.

Pre-ovulation

O Oestrogen increases leading to the development of the egg follicles, stimulation of breast tissue and the uterine wall.

Ovulation

O At ovulation time (around day 12–16) usually just one egg is released from one of your fallopian tubes (they tend to alternate each month).

O You will notice a change in your discharge around this time. You will most likely feel very wet, and your underwear will be damp from the discharge which is clear and stretchy like egg white. It can often feel like you have just got your period. You will most likely feel sexier. If you are wanting to get pregnant, now's the time!

- The egg becomes a *corpus luteum* producing both oestrogen and progesterone in preparation for fertilisation.

Pre-menstrual

- The pre-menstrual stage can last for six to ten days before bleeding starts.

- If fertilisation does not occur the *corpus luteum* degenerates and the levels of progesterone and oestrogen both fall.

- This change in hormones can lead to PMS symptoms.

- Most women have a second window of sexual excitement either just before or during menstruation.

- There is a biological need for increased REM (dreaming) sleep from day 25 onwards.

- Most women report that their sleep is affected by their menstrual cycle, being worst in the three days before bleeding and continuing into the heaviest bleeding days.

Many women have regular cycles of around 28 days, though others might have cycles of varying lengths (14–40 days), and periods of varying lengths (3–7 days). What is most important is that you know what 'normal' is for you.

Our cycles can be impacted by stress or illness. If you have had a stressful month, don't be surprised if your period is late.

Some women naturally have shorter or longer cycles their whole lives, however if:

- your periods are very irregular
- you have a lot of mid-cycle spotting

○ your period is very light (pale pink and watery)

○ it is extremely heavy

○ it contains lots of clots

○ PMS symptoms are incapacitating

○ you are struggling to conceive

I do recommend that you visit a practitioner—both your doctor, and perhaps an acupuncturist or herbalist—to help you to establish a rhythm. This is especially important if you are wanting to chart your cycles either to avoid pregnancy or to find out your peak fertile time.

Irregular cycles and the other issues mentioned can be symptomatic of an underlying health issue that needs to be addressed.

Menstruation and breastfeeding

There is little common knowledge about the interaction between menstruation and lactation, perhaps because at the time when much of the scientific research on menstruation was happening in the West, breastfeeding levels were at their lowest since humans' emergence on the planet.

○ Prolactin, the major hormone which enables breastfeeding, suppresses fertility. This natural pause to the cycles is called lactational amenorrhea. Some women use this as a contraceptive technique, known as the Lactational Amenorrhea Method (LAM). It is only recommended whilst the baby is being nursed exclusively, is under the age of six months and menstrual bleeding has not returned. For more see www.waba.org.my/resources/lam/

○ Extended periods of lactational amenorrhea result in

lower rates of breast, ovarian and endometrial cancers.

O Fertility may reappear anything from four weeks after birth to over three years. With mothers who breastfeed exclusively, it is usually over six months, and often over a year.

O The first periods may occur without ovulation, but equally fertility might reappear without menstruation, and with no obvious signs to alert you.

O It is completely possible to conceive whilst breastfeeding. However, some women might need to cut down feeds or stop feeding altogether to ensure a return to full fertility.

O Breastfeeding affects the vaginal secretions (due to low oestrogen) so mucus charting can be ineffective. Be sure to use your temperature if you are charting your fertility naturally.

O Readjusting to your menstrual cycles after pregnancy and feeding can be a gradual process, with periods taking a while to establish their regular rhythm.

O Return to menstruation can be accompanied by emotional upheaval including: grief, depression, exhaustion. It may also bring renewed energy, a rise in your libido and a feeling of 'being back to yourself'.

Menopause

The most powerful force in the world is a menopausal woman with zest.

Margaret Mead

Menopause refers to the last menstrual period. It occurs at some point between 40 and 55 years old, with the average being 51 years. It is considered conclusive when you have 12 months without a period.

○ *Pre*-menopause can last ten years. During this time the ovaries gradually stop maturing eggs and releasing large amounts of hormones.

○ *Peri*-menopause refers to the few years before and one year after the final period where symptoms are usually apparent. Progesterone levels begin to decline. Although you may have seemingly normal menstrual periods, they begin to occur without ovulation (inovulatory cycles). Without adequate progesterone, oestrogen becomes the dominant hormone.

○ This leads to the onset of well-known menopausal symptoms: hot flushes, night sweats, mood swings, insomnia, vaginal dryness, lack of sex-drive, weight gain and irregular periods. And to lesser-known ones: breast tenderness, headaches and heavier, prolonged menstrual flows.

○ Post-menopausal women need to take extra care of their bone and cardiovascular health.

○ Due to the increasing amount of oestrogen-mimicking, hormone disrupting chemicals in our foods, the water supply, plastics and other products we use on a daily basis, women are experiencing oestrogen dominance much earlier in life than in the past. It's now not unusual to notice symptoms of menopause in your late thirties. This does not necessarily mean that you are about to experience menopause. Have your hormone levels checked, and ask a practitioner about supplementing with natural progesterone.

Just as our culture demonises menstruation and birth, menopause has also been simultaneously silenced, trivialised and made a terrifying prospect. During her medical residency, Dr Eve Agee noticed that women with persistent menstrual problems also tend to suffer more during menopause. A fact which on the surface seems self-evident, but because of the way our medical system specialises so heavily, womb issues may be dealt with by a number of different specialists over the course of a woman's life: from menarche, through childbirth and menopause, and the dots may not be joined. Therefore it is key to heal your menstrual cycles now, whilst you still have them, so that your transition through menopause is a smoother ride.

THE WISDOM OF OUR CYCLES

By being true to all sides of your nature, you acknowledge that you can be self-confident, active and strong, that you can nurture without being weak, that you can be wild and instinctual as well as calm and reasoning, and that you have a beautiful darkness within, a depth beyond the mundane world.

Miranda Gray, *Red Moon*

We have mentioned our 'cycles' quite a lot now in passing. And sometimes we forget the meaning of the word. A cycle is the basic unit of life: birth, growth, transformation, decline and death, followed once again by birth. It is a circular, repeating journey. A process of expansion and contraction, which is echoed in the pulsations of the womb, the beating of our hearts, the in and out of our breath. Cycles can be observed in every life form on the planet, in the seasons and the phases of the moon. Our menstrual cycles connect our female bodies directly to nature.

Our cycles ensure that we do not live static lives. Instead they demand that we live dynamically, constantly exploring the different gifts of feminine power that each portion of our cycle holds. Part of learning the art of being a woman is learning to honour each element of our cycles and ourselves.

The menstrual cycle is, in the words of Alexandra Pope, '*our inner guidance system, initiating us into and anointing us with ever deepening revelation and wisdom.*' In the next few chapters I will share the ways in which we can tune into this guidance system, and grow in our own cyclical wisdom.

So let us delve deeper into what it means to be a cycling woman. Let us examine the intricate interweaving of our bodies, hormones and psyches which make us the women we are.

Dancing in the dark

Our menstrual cycle takes us each month on a journey between the light and dark in a spiral dance. Each month we get another opportunity to dance in a different way, to interact with our rhythms and tune in through our bodies. When we are unskilled or unprepared, we may stumble, falling over our own feet and everything that lies in our path.

But as we gain confidence in ourselves and sense our own rhythm we begin to dance to our own tune. We sense when the energy shifts and rather than resist, we follow its lead.

> *The movements of the cycle are like the breath catching, like the snagging of threads in a garment. A sudden shift in gear, a cloud scudding across the sun, a small irritation, a distraction. Quiet, subtle, demanding your attention. Tripping you into different realities, perspectives and understandings. Breaking the mould of the cultural mind set. Stopping you from becoming an endless doing machine. Reminding you of yourself and making you sensitive to the world.*
> **Alexandra Pope *The Wild Genie: The Healing Power of Menstruation***

A cycle

As a way of illustrating the dynamic journey of the menstrual cycle, what better way than to share with you one of my own cycles? Rather than impersonal diagrams I present you with a personal narrative in the hope that you might recognise elements and patterns, which had previously gone unnoticed in your own life.

Day One

For the past couple of days I have known that my moon time is approaching. It has felt like a storm is building—internal pressure growing until I felt I would burst. I have been irritable, on edge, my belly has felt fat and blobby. I hate my clothes and my body. I just want to be left alone.

The moon has gone and the nights are really dark. As I was putting the children to bed, I wanted them to hurry up and be gone. I found them too energetic. I needed the smooth, slow darkness of my own mind. I wanted to be alone with my thoughts, to sink into them like a warm bath. Once they were in bed I felt drawn to my journal and silence.

My moon time blood feels like sweet relief. Like the storm clouds breaking and the rain pouring down after a drought. It takes all my energy with it. I feel hollow and empty, like I have nothing left to say or give, and it feels like the world is pouring out of me. I lie or sit all the time, with no desire to go for a walk or do anything energetic. I just need to be quiet and alone in this dreamlike state.

Day Two

Last night I dreamt of blood and terrifying strange men. My dreams feel as real as waking life at this stage: vivid and powerful. They stay with me all day.

My bleeding is still heavy, but I am hit with a surge of energy. If I am not careful I quickly overdo it. It doesn't take much to make me exhausted—rather like during pregnancy. I have to remember to pace myself otherwise I will be pretty much bed-ridden with exhaustion for the next couple of days.

Days Three and Four

My bleeding is easing up little by little, and as it does my energy returns more.

Day Five

With my bleeding virtually gone I feel back to myself and renewed. I feel the need to purify, to cleanse my body. I always have a sacred bath at this point, a literal washing away of the smell and feel of menstruation. It is a time for sloughing off dead skin and old feelings, to break fresh and clean into the new cycle. I don't like having baths during my moon time so it always feels like a real treat to have one to mark its end. I luxuriate with a rose candle, bubble bath and steam rising up.

Days Six to Nine

It feels so good to be more energetic. I want to be out in the world. Ideas start to flow. . . and the energy to see them through. My emotions feel clear and fresh. My libido starts to rise again. My heart energy rises, I want to be close and affectionate, where only three days ago I desired nothing more than to be alone and untouched. It feels so good to be alive.

Days Ten to Twelve

My energy is soaring. With the clear flow of my ovulatory phase I celebrate with my sexual being. This is the fertile time, when all my children were conceived. It is a time for creativity—with body and soul. I have so many projects that I want to start right now! I invite friends round for an impromptu party and we stay up chatting till late.

Days Thirteen to Sixteen

Full moon is here and with it my ovulation—I feel deeply connected to the openness of the moon. I feel lit up. I also feel a little crampy at this time of the month. I go for a walk on the beach and watch the moon rise over the sea, soaking up the bright moonlight, and give thanks for all I have.

My energy feels clear and flowing, I am focused and creative and have huge amounts of energy—I could take over the world right now! I enjoy nourishing myself and my family, and entertaining friends. I fill my fridge and freezer with meals to sustain us when I no longer feel like cooking.

Days Seventeen to Nineteen

I notice my energy levels starting to lessen—I am between the worlds, neither ovulatory nor pre-menstrual. I feel on edge, I check my calendar to see when I am due ... surely it can't be that long.

Days Twenty to Twenty-three

I feel like I am starting to sink down. Things become more of an effort. I notice my patience getting shorter and I get upset more easily.

Days Twenty-four to Twenty-seven

A tireder, heavier energy emerges, I feel sluggish, and everything is an effort. I am spaced out and can't concentrate on things which earlier in the month I would have flown through. I feel tired. Really tired. I bawl in front of a soppy TV program. I growl about my husband's imperfections in my head. I snap impatiently at the kids in the morning rush, then burst into tears straight afterwards. I am craving sugar. Nothing feels right. I would really just like to curl up like a cat in a cosy chair in front of a roaring fire, and not be bothered. I feel like I'm coming down with flu: tired, aching bones and belly, and hot and cold flushes. If I let myself have time alone, if I let myself really express what is wrong and let it out, I feel much better.

Day Twenty-eight

I need to be nurtured. I need warming food, a blanket round my shoulders and to curl up in bed early. So I do. I put on a nourishing women's summit broadcast and soak in gentle feminine wisdom. My absolute *need* for chocolate reaches a crescendo in the week before my period. It is so strong: a dark, comforting warmth that soothes me. It drives me nuts that I can't eat it because of migraines.

I have also noticed that in the few hours before my period I suddenly become sexually alert and responsive, just as I do at ovulation. I am alive, let's celebrate with sex! And then these feelings totally disappear for the next five days.

AND YOU?

How much of this sounds familiar to you from your own cycle?

And where does your cycle differ?

The archetypes

Our cycles have four major phases, which can be interpreted as corresponding to the four main female archetypes (or energy patterns) and stages of life.

The Virgin/Maiden

The Virgin self emerges after the menstrual bleeding has stopped, and the fresh new womb lining grows.

She is full of innocence, energy and potential. She feels good in her body—flirtatious, sexy and lighter after the dark days of her blood time. Her ability to conceive and gestate are just emerging and are still unproven. At this point in her cycle she feels free from her menstrual pull—she is a virgin in the traditional sense of the word—a woman unto herself.

The Mother

The time of ovulation and possible conception is represented by the mother who has the ability to nurture new life. Her fertile womb space is warm and soft. At this time a woman tends to feel loving and enjoys giving of herself fully, either by becoming a mother to a child, or in her career, creativity or home-making. Ovulation symbolises the ability to give and sustain life and the full flourishing of a woman's life.

The Enchantress/Wild Woman

The pre-menstrual stage is a descent from the light, outward stage of our cycle and into the dark, inner stage. Progesterone and oestrogen dance together to create dynamic swings. The Wild Woman dances a magical path between huge bouts of creativity and emotional storms. In time you learn how to harness this powerful energy, knowing when to destroy, how to express your righteous anger, and when to go within and reflect.

The Crone/Wise Woman

The Crone emerges during the late pre-menstrual and bleeding time. She can be a Wise Woman or a destructive Witch depending on how she handles this time. Her mood darkens and she becomes pulled inward, becoming quieter, more reflective and more in touch with the dream time. She is less 'in the world' and in need of more rest. She has no need to please others, and lives according to her own inner wisdom and guidance. This time has many gifts for a woman and her community, if she can learn to retreat and allow her visions to emerge from her depths, trusting her wisdom.

OOO

We live in a culture which worships the Virgin, her nubile body and budding sexuality. One which side-lines the Mother, not celebrating or honouring the acts of gestation, birth and childrearing. A culture which fears the power of the Enchantress, which turns away from the wisdom of the elders and does not know the value of reflection and dreams.

In order to reclaim our full selves, to integrate each of these aspects through which we pass over the course of our lives, we must first learn to embrace them though our cycles.

We need to take time to honour the part of ourselves that mothers and nurtures; the part of us that yearns to be girlish, free and self-defined; the wise woman who watches in the wings full of wisdom and the erotic enchantress who can bewitch and create magic. Our cycles allow us to take on these roles, to live these hidden parts of our psyches.

Our cycling nature gives us constant teasing tastes of the whole gamut of womanhood, and our life cycle, month after month. It also ensures that we deal with emotions which we might otherwise avoid: anger, sadness, conflict, grief and eroticism.

We are always much more complex, much wiser than we give ourselves credit for; our potential much greater than we dare to hope or dream.

Creating your archetypes

Many esoteric and mystical traditions consider the womb to be a crucible of creativity: sexual, reproductive and artistic. It has been identified with the 'holy grail' of myth and legend, a magical, life-giving cup of rejuvenation and knowledge. Throughout the book I will offer suggestions of how you might tap into your innate, embodied creativity in your womb space.

If the archetypes in this chapter resonate with you, then why not bring them to life for yourself? The following exercise will help you to integrate their different energies further into your life.

The exercise is divided into a couple of stages—the first step is connecting internally with the energies and emotions connected to each archetype, then visualising these in your mind's eye in terms of colour and symbol, before representing them creatively.

You do not need to be a professional artist to have a go. It is about building your understanding of the different energies as represented by the archetypal characters. Your intention needs to be expressing the basic energy of each phase of the cycle—your representations do not need to be 'perfect', they are your unique expressions of your personal understanding. If you really, really freak out at the idea of putting brush to paper, then just do this as an active visualisation, taking yourself through the steps in your head.

Take what you learn from it and apply it into your physical experience of your cycle—dress in the colours that resonate with you at that time of the month, move in the way that you associate with that archetype, integrate your intuitive understanding of each archetypal phase into your daily life.

Materials

First you need to choose the art materials that you wish to work with—something which allows quick work is better, as this is responsive, intuitive work—so if you choose paints, then I recommend acrylics, gouache or watercolours, not oils. Clay feels lovely between the fingers for a tactile, sensual experience. Pastels (chalky ones, not oil pastels) are great for beginning creatives as they are soft and forgiving. You can cover a lot of space quickly with them and if you are unhappy with something you can rub it out with your finger. For exercise one I recommend that you choose one medium (i.e. paint, pastel, clay) to create the whole series, so that you have a complete cycle and you can see how the energy alters the identical materials.

Set up your space

Make it somewhere where you can work undisturbed. Or if you are working alongside your children (as I often do) make it clear that you are working on your special project and they are working on theirs. Ensure that they are settled with their work before you begin.

Have all the materials you will need to hand and make sure surfaces are protected. Switch off your phone. You may want to light incense or smudge the space with sage. Perhaps have some music which feels sacred to you—choose it according to the energy you are working with. This project can take place over the course of a month. Or it could be a moon time project.

Centre yourself

Before you start your work, centre yourself with a few deep, mindful breaths. Place your hands on your belly, breathe in and out, bringing your attention to your womb. Bring your attention to where in your cycle you are. Have to hand the Integrated Menstrual Chart (see p46) as a reference.

Visualisation

Concentrate on the archetype and answer the following questions instinctively, without excessive rationalisation and logical thought. There are no right or wrong answers—this is your interpretation. You can jot down your ideas if it helps:

- What colours do you associate with this archetype?
- What natural forms?
- What objects?
- What physical posture?
- What energy levels?
- What symbols?
- Where does she live?
- With whom?
- How does she wear her hair?
- What clothes does she wear?

○ How does she move?

○ What animal might she be?

○ What element do you associate with her?

Exercise one—full series

In this exercise you will create a series of four pictures, each worked quickly and intuitively to express the archetypes. You will need four pieces of paper, one for each archetype.

You will be starting with the Virgin/Maiden. Pause for a moment, settling into your body. Hold the key words which resonate with you about her in your mind as you work, keeping in mind the season, her element etc.

Then pick a colour and start to work, quickly and intuitively.

After ten minutes move onto the Mother. Again, sit with the archetype for a few moments first, welcoming her energy into your body. After another ten minutes move on to the Enchantress and finally the Wise Woman.

Step back and behold them, now you have the series, see if there is anything that you want to highlight about their similarities or differences. In this way you will produce a series of pictures in under an hour. Finish by taking a few minutes to write in your journal about any insight that came to you in the process of creating these archetypes.

Exercise two—cycle project

You can also work more deeply, throughout the course of a cycle. For this variation you commit to one hour (roughly) at each phase in your cycle. Still yourself and tune into the energy that is coursing around your body at that moment. Really feel it. And then take that onto the paper. Paint or draw yourself in this phase—what colours best express your mood, are you dynamic or still, what posture feels right to you?

Exercise three—branching out

Another time, perhaps you will choose to drum, dance, write monologues or poems, make a quilt or puppet, a piece of jewellery, or a self-portrait photograph for each different phase of your cycle.

Giving expression to these energies is fulfilling and insightful and can only lead you to greater self-knowledge.

If you are a professional artist, it might also lead you into some deep, personal works which profoundly touch the women who see them.

AND YOU?

Have you ever thought how your creativity is connected to your womb?

How much does your creativity express your experience of living in a female body?

PUTTING THE MOON BACK INTO MENSTRUATION

Everything that flows moves in rhythm with the moon. She rules the water element on Earth. She pulls the ocean's tides, the weather, female reproductive cycles and the life fluids of plants, animals and people. She influences the mood swings of mind, body, behavior and emotion.

WeMoon Diary

That the 28-day menstrual cycle correlates closely with the moon's cycle, as well as the fact that women living in close proximity cycle together, are some of the more mysterious elements of the menstrual cycle which science and the world at large seem to have little interest in. But once women are aware of this, it adds an extra dimension to their appreciation of the intricate sensitivity of their bodies to the natural world around them. It is truly remarkable that the pull of a distant astronomical body has such an impact on our own small selves.

Our connection to the moon might seem at first glance to be a rather esoteric belief, but science now backs it up.

A growing understanding of ecology and feedback systems has led us to see that every living organism is in constant contact with its surrounding environment and continuously influenced by it.

We tend to think that our biological rhythms are independent of the environment, but many of them were originally acquired through interaction with the outside world. It is not by chance that women's menstrual cycles and the moon's phase correspond, any more than it is coincidence that all people have built in diurnal rhythms of approximately the same length. At one time moonlight and sunlight actually controlled such functions directly but through evolution these rhythms have become incorporated into our biological systems.

Prof. Kerstin Uvnas Moberg, *The Oxytocin Factor: Tapping the Hormone of Calm, Love and Healing*

There is increasing evidence from research on people and animals alike that the destruction of biological rhythms has implications for an organism's health and general well-being. Our bodies were born on this Earth, programmed by our genes and enculturation to be tied to the sun's daily rhythms for waking and sleeping—and the moon for our menstrual cycles and subconscious life processes.

It has been proven that the full moon has a strong negative impact on the quality of sleep, regardless of whether the moon is visible or not.

Many professionals attest to the very real influence of the moon on human behaviour in their work. Teachers will tell you that their students are more unruly and 'wired' at full moon. Many police forces in the UK and US ensure higher staffing levels on full moons, in anticipation of extra violence. Casualty admissions often spike. And midwives are aware that the full moon seems to trigger labour in many pregnant women.

The influence of the full moon has been observed for centuries and is where we get the word *lunatic* from—meaning somebody who experiences temporary or heightened insanity at full moon.

Current research shows an increase in schizophrenic and epileptic episodes at full moon time.

We are not the only species influenced by the moon—corals spawn, wolves howl and turtles lay eggs at the full moon. Tides are higher. Traditionally farmers planted and harvested by the moon's cycles as well, and many still use these principles to guide their growing practices.

Phases of the moon

The moon is constantly changing in appearance—her shape and size determined by her position relative to the sun that illuminates her. Not only does she change in appearance, but also when she rises and sets. The moon rises in the east and sets in the west each day.

The moon has a cycle of approximately 29.5 days. On months where there are two full moons in a calendar month it is called a *blue* moon—hence the phrase 'once in a blue moon' as it is a reasonably unusual occurrence. A *super* moon is when the moon is at its closest point to Earth and appears noticeably larger in the sky—this is considered to amplify its influence upon people and nature.

The following is a simplified version of the moon's phases and the energetic properties of each.

Full Moon

Full moons rise at sunset and set at dawn. They are energising—sometimes in a good way, at others creating agitation, making sleep and relaxation hard. Full moons are a time to harvest and sow, a time to entertain and celebrate, to work late and create wholeheartedly.

Each full moon has its own special name and characteristics.

For example the full moon which falls at some time in mid-August through to mid-September is called the *Harvest* moon—it tends to seem particularly golden and full, and its light was used to harvest by.

Waning moon

Waning means getting smaller. When the moon reaches its halfway point (the last quarter moon, which rises around midnight) there is a sense of balance, tension or transition. It continues getting smaller each night, until it is completely dark.

The dark moon or new moon

For a couple of days the moon is almost invisible, it is a time of darkness. The moon is in shadow and rises before dawn and sets with the sun. Many traditions use this as a time of inwardness, reflection, visioning and setting intentions for the month ahead. It is a time of new beginnings, a seeming pause in the darkness before its journey back to fullness again.

Waxing moon

The moon gets a little bigger and brighter each night, moving through the *crescent* moon—the moon of story-books, the small sliver which speaks of hope, new life, magic. At halfway (the first quarter) again there is a sense of transition or balance, the moon is visible in the afternoon and sets in the evening.

Many cultures run on lunar calendars, but ours is solar. To learn more about the moon's phases, get yourself a calendar or diary with the lunar cycle in it. Make a conscious effort to check the sky every day, and mark the days of your cycle onto your calendar so you can see how your menstrual cycle and the phases of the moon interact.

Our personal moon cycles

The most common menstrual pattern is to bleed on the dark moon and to ovulate at full moon, this is known as the **White Moon Cycle.**

Before the advent of electric light in the late nineteenth century, women's ovulation was primarily activated by their hormonal response to the brightness of the full moon at night. In our modern era however, street lighting, domestic electric lighting, artificial hormones, pollutants and stress have contributed to women's cycles being more staggered throughout the month, with some bleeding rather than ovulating at full moon (known as the **Red Moon Cycle**), and many others unconnected to the moon's cycles at all. Women who have charted their cycles and experienced menstruation at dark and full moon report feeling more 'in flow' and 'attuned to themselves' when they bleed on the dark moon.

In the wonderful book *Alchemy for Women*, Penelope Shuttle makes brief reference to the **Wise Woman Cycle**—a menstrual pattern which alternates every three months or so between White Moon and Red Moon Cycles.

This has been my pattern, since getting my moon time back after having my third child. It is slightly disorientating feeling—one month being in sync with the energetic pull of the moon—bleeding on the dark moon, feeling naturally introspective and in need of retreat, and then ovulating and having high energy at the same time as the moon is at its fullest (and the children are at their most hyper!) Menstruation at full moon three to four months later is quite a different dynamic, and the full moon energy makes resting harder, but acts to strengthen the visioning and creative powers which come to the fore during this part of our cycle. This constantly shifting cycle within the cycle, means you are always kept on your toes, having to adapt. It gives new insights into your own cycle and the moon's cycle, and the subtleties of their various combinations.

There is little information available about the Wise Woman Cycle, and so I asked a number of the leading women in the field of menstruation, most of whom had not come across it either! I loved Sophia Style's insight:

After ten years of sharing our menstrual cycles in women's circles, I have also seen this pattern repeated many, many times, and in myself (although not always as clear as every three months!)

My feeling is that the dark moon and the full moon are powerful magnets for our menstruation and that our moon time, for most women, tends to journey from one to another. It feels very different either way (the specific insights and experiences also vary from woman to woman from what we have shared). To experience both kinds of cycles so regularly, and the different wisdom that each brings (from deeply inward to intensely open and all kinds of permutations in between) in a conscious way, is no doubt a Wise Woman Cycle.

Celebrating full moon

Cultures around the world celebrate the full moon and its vibrant energies in different ways—from full moon parties on Thai beaches to Jewish family feasts.

Whilst celebrations tied to the moon are often associated with Pagan and Wiccan traditions, more mainstream religions also use the moon to guide their feast days. In the Christian tradition the date of Easter changes each year, according to where the full moon falls. The Jewish calendar is rooted in the cycles of the moon, Rosh Chodesh is marked each new moon and Yom Kippur Katan is celebrated the day before, as a day of fasting and penitence in preparation for the new month ahead. The Islamic festival of Ramadan begins on the day after new moon, and ends on the sighting of the next month's crescent moon.

Calendars in many Asian countries are lunar based. The most important Buddhist celebrations, Vesak, Sangha Day and Dhamma Day are all celebrated on the full moon. In Hinduism the moon cycles are considered very powerful, and devotees will fast on both the full and new moons of each month. Diwali is celebrated on the new moon and Holi on the last full moon of winter.

Creating your own full moon celebrations

Spending time out in the bright light of the full moon is a magical experience, even for the most cynical of us. If you are looking to realign your menstrual cycle with the moon's cycle so that you have a White Moon Cycle, exposure to the full moon light can have a very powerful effect. Many women who have tried the 'lunar realignment' of their cycles have contacted me reporting great success.

For those of you who enjoy deepening your physical connection to the moon, here are some of my favourite energising full moon activities.

○ Full moon circles that gather to celebrate the full moon—often for women only, the participants dance and co-create rituals and ceremony.

○ Moon bathe! Go outside and feel the electric glow of moonlight and chill on your skin, take your shoes off, perhaps even your top in mid-summer! Feel the dew beneath your feet. Put a blanket on the grass if it is damp and lie on your back, looking up at the moon, the stars and the vast expanse of the heavens.

○ Celebrate the full moon and the rise in your fertility and desire with your partner—or alone. Dance together, make love, have a moonlight picnic and frolic in the dew.

O   Enjoy a sensual moonlight swim or moonlight stroll.

O   Open your curtains and sleep in the bright moon light.

O   As you walk through your house turning off your lights before you go to bed, take a moment to gaze up at the moon through your window, and allow yourself to breathe and be fully present.

O   Try Moon Essences which help you attune to the qualities of the full moon energy—these can be purchased, or try steeping herbs or crystals in water in the light of the full moon.

New moon celebrations

The new moon is a time of sowing seeds and visioning what we desire in the month ahead.

O   Create a red tent or moon lodge and sit in circle with other women.

O   Attend a sweat lodge.

O   Take time to sink into your intuition using practices that you love.

O   Vision your month ahead in your journal as a quiet, introspective practice.

A moon time myth

Other cultures and other times have had different understandings of the female body, its innate rhythms and wisdom. Other cultures have honoured the menstrual blood as wise, the moon as a powerful force and the ability to give birth as a miracle.

The following story is one from the Native American tradition, retold by one of their elders, Nicholas Noblewolf. It tells of their understanding of the significance of a woman's moon time, and how it should be respected by all, as a precious gift from Grandmother Moon.

A long time ago, women did as they do now—they held the family, they held the power (life-force) for the family, they held the happiness and joy, they held the sorrow and disappointments. After time, the negative emotions and heartache that the women took upon themselves on behalf of their families would begin to weigh them down. The women would become sick and finally, could no longer take on the burdens of the family. Yet the nature to do so had been imbued into them by Creator.

One day, a woman was out in the forest, crying because the burden had become so great, when Raven heard her and asked, 'Mother, why do you cry?'

The woman responded, 'I love my family so very much. I hold my family in my heart and soul, but the pains of life have filled me up. I can no longer help my family. I can no longer take their burdens from them. I just don't know what to do.'

Raven responded, 'I understand the pain you feel, as I feel it also. I will go and ask Grandmother Ocean if she knows what to do.' So Raven flew to the ocean and shared with Grandmother the plight of the women.

Grandmother Ocean responded, 'If the women will come to me, I will wash their pain from them, but this won't help the ones who are far away. Let me ask my sister, Grandmother Moon, if she can help.'

So Grandmother Ocean spoke to her sister of the women's plight. Grandmother Moon responded, 'I am the power of the feminine. I will send into the women, my sisters, your waters carrying my power. Once every moon cycle, you shall come into the women through me and purify them.' And, she did this. So ever since then, every woman has a time each moon cycle when she embodies the power of the moon and flows the cleansing of the ocean. We call this the woman's time of the moon, or moon-time.

It is each woman's responsibility to take the time when she is in her time of the moon to purify. It is the responsibility of the men to give the women the opportunity to do so.

Nicholas Noble Wolf, www.nicholasnoblewolf.com

This story was taken from an article first published in *Sacred Hoop* magazine 2000. It is republished here with the author's permission.

CHARTING YOUR CYCLE

Our bodies are in constant, rhythmic change, but because so much of this is happening beneath our waking consciousness, we can feel out of control, or 'all at sea'. When we begin to notice the pattern of these cycles, their repetitive nature, their connection to nature beyond us, we can begin to feel not like victims unprepared for the weather, but like adventurers of days gone by, who navigate by nature—the pull of the tides, the placing of the stars and the gathering storm clouds.

Often we can feel overwhelmed and confused by the seeming turbulence of our bodies and unpredictability of our moods. If this is you, then I thoroughly recommend charting your cycle for a few months, to get a deeper understanding of how your body and moods change throughout your cycle. This will help you to navigate your life from an inner stability, and an awareness of your own unique ebb and flow.

There are many ways to keep track of your cycle:

○ marking the expected date of your period in your diary

○ using an app on your phone

○ charting symptoms for fertility awareness (see next chapter)—to aid conception or contraception

○ charting symptoms in a journal for healing PMS

○ keeping a moon diary—where you chart your symptoms alongside the moon's phases

O using a moon dial

O or perhaps a moon bracelet, often called a mala or lunar time piece

(For stockists of all of these see the Resources section at the end of the book.)

I have been charting my cycle for many years, in different ways:

O scientifically as a natural contraceptive method, noting the changes in discharge. (NB this produced two surprise babies for us!)

O to give insight into my PMS, noting what foods, events and parts of my cycle were in need of attention and healing

O directly into my diary, both with moon cycles and without, to see what impact and correlation the moon has on my cycles

O my dreams and how they connect to my cycle

O sometimes in a more descriptive form, as you saw earlier

Each method reveals insight into your changing, cyclical self, by recording the tiny details which we tend to overlook, or if we do notice them we forget exactly when they occurred. Charting shows us physiological and emotional patterns over the course of the month, and makes us more mindful of our eating, self-care regime, energy levels and fertility.

OOO

AND YOU?

Have you charted before? Which aspects worked, and which didn't?

What kind of charting calls to you?

What do you want to understand more about? PMS, fertility, your moods?

Using a moon dial

A moon dial gives a great reminder of the repetitive, cyclical nature of your menstrual cycle and is particularly helpful for visual learners. The moon dial can be an interactive journey of discovery of oneself in relation to the moon's own cycles. Through exploring and aligning these cycles we can create liberation by balancing our whole being.

With your moon dial you can:

O   note the phase of the moon relative to your cycle

O   place the date next to each day to keep track easily

O   note physical symptoms, general health, energy levels, activity and dreams

See my video on The Happy Womb on how to use a moon dial. There are a few different versions that I have come across—see the Resources section at the back of the book for stockists.

If you can't get or make a dial, why not start a moon diary? Each day of your cycle note down a couple of words about your emotional state, energy levels and any physical symptoms to begin to see the course of your moon journey that your hormones and body are following.

Dream charting

Another key way to gain insight into our menstrual cycles is through dream charting. This is something I learned from the fabulous book, *Alchemy for Women* by Penelope Shuttle. I highly recommend seeking out a copy to learn more about it.

It was a revelation to me that our dreams alter according to our menstrual cycles. Images that might occur at ovulation include: a clear river, babies, small animals, eggs, balls, images of pregnancy or birth, erotic dreams. Whereas dreams that tend to occur approaching menstruation include: blood, red images (red flowers, red clothes), being wounded or bleeding, also dark haunting dreams of death, being pursued by a dark man. The threshold points, when we move from ovulatory to pre-menstrual and pre-menstrual to bleeding are often accompanied by particularly powerful and vivid dreams. What is even more fascinating is that our menstrual cycles can affect our partner's dreams!

Charting our dreams—writing down what we remember of them as soon as we awaken—gives us a profound insight into the crossovers between our bodies and minds, and our subconscious world. Often when reflecting on these dreams we can find wisdom for our waking lives.

Integrated menstrual chart

On the following pages you will find the biological, archetypal, spiritual and emotional cycle wisdom I have compiled in this book in a simple chart format, condensing the ideas into a clear reference tool.

You could photocopy it and keep in your journal or pin it on the wall by your desk as a reminder of your ever-changing self. You could illustrate it, colour it or laminate it. . .

It is yours to use in the way that supports you best. My deepest wish is that it will guide you in your journey of self-discovery.

You will find a full-colour version to download for yourself or share with your friends on my website www.thehappywomb.com

	PRE-OVULATORY	OVULATORY
MOON PHASE	Waxing	Full
ARCHETYPE	Virgin/Maiden	Mother
SEASON	Spring	Summer
ELEMENT	Air	Earth
LIGHT	Lightening	Full bright light
LENGTH	9 days	5 days
HORMONE	Oestrogen	Rising oestrogen and progesterone.
PHYSICAL	Egg follicle ripening—stimulating breast and womb.	Egg released from ovary into fallopian tube, becomes *corpus luteum*. Uterine wall built up in preparation for fertilisation.
VAGINAL DISCHARGE	Sticky/none	Clear and stretchy, like egg white. Very wet feeling.
EMOTION	Calm, open, dynamic, clear, energetic, enthusiastic, able to cope with irritations.	Loving, nurturing, nourishing, sustaining, energised, connected.
ENERGY	Rising dynamic—growing outward.	Full, sustaining—losing sense of self in work or mothering.

Pre-menstrual	Menstrual
Waning	Dark
Enchantress/Wild Woman	Crone/Wise Woman
Autumn	Winter
Fire	Water
Darkening	Dark
9 days	5 days
Falling oestrogen and progesterone.	Progesterone
Transition time.	Womb lining breaks down and released from uterus.
None/blobby, thick and yellow	Bleeding—starting out bright red, becoming browner towards the end.
Creative, emotional, sensitive, angry.	Introspective, dreamy, sensitive, intuitive, spiritually connected.
Waning dynamic—destructive, descending inward.	Reflective, slow, containing, internalised, spiritual.

	PRE-OVULATORY	OVULATORY
LIBIDO	Rising, carefree.	Full, horny, height of libidinous desire around full moon/ovulation.
PHYSICAL FEELING	Energetic	Perhaps ovulatory pain/cramping, sometimes mid-cycle spotting, food cravings, horny, sensitive breasts.
OUTWARD ACTION	Start projects—clear visioning and energy raising. Fresh start. Organise and prioritise. Clear out—spring cleaning. Catch up with things that have slipped during menstruation.	Work hard, love well—birth creative projects, stay up late! Harmony with nature and other mothers. Receptive to other's input.
RELATIONSHIPS	Easy-going, trusting, out-going.	Loving, giving, nurturing. Reach out to friends, children, family and partner.
KEY WORDS	New beginnings, dynamic, exuberance, self-confident.	Fertility, radiating, caring, nurturing, committed.
AFFIRMATION	I step forward in action with a lightness of heart.	I embrace my life with love and generate beauty around me.

PRE-MENSTRUAL	MENSTRUAL
Peaks and troughs—can be very intense.	Often a sexual peak just before bleeding occurs, or just after. Little desire during menstruation.
Lowered immune system. Towards the end: cramping, back ache, bloating, tiredness, tender breasts, sugar and carbohydrate cravings, hostility, mood swings.	Greater need for rest and dreaming sleep. Cramping, back ache, migraine, faintness, exhaustion, tearfulness.
Finish up projects. Begin to reflect and assess. Take action dealing with issues and problems. Turn your focus to inner-directed creative projects and listen deeply to your intuition.	Retreat, dream time. Only do what is essential. Do not take on any new projects. Delay important decisions or stressful appointments. Slow down, tune in deeply to your intuition and rest well.
Needs to balance dynamic interactions with others, with focused, energised creative time alone.	Desires to be alone or in quiet communion with other women—does not want to be around men and children!
Magical, witchy, destructive, intuitive.	Darkness, wisdom, gestation, stillness, vision.
I use the sword of my intolerance to cut deep and true. I keep hold of my vision and manifest it.	I sink into my depths and listen to my dreams.

OUR FERTILITY

Fertility spans the arc of womanhood—menarche-menstruation–birth–menopause. Whether we intend to birth or not, have gone through menopause or not, fertility is the arc of womanhood.

Lorraine Ferrier, natural fertility expert

Our periods are often looked at in isolation from our fertility and feelings about fertility. In my own personal experience, and that of women that I know, how we feel about getting pregnant majorly impacts our attitudes towards our moon time and our bodies. It shifts and changes according to where we are in our fertility journeys.

Our culture has a rather warped view of fertility: it's considered a bad thing. . . until some point in your thirties, where you then 'should' have babies (the right amount, in the right way, with the right partner and spacing and not too many) before a cut off period where you definitely 'should not' have them.

Let's have a look at the archetypes of our fertility, and then at how we can build our fertility awareness.

Fertility and the four phases of womanhood

Virgin

For younger women who dread the inconvenience of pregnancy, and just desire to be free and easy in their bodies, like they were as a pre-teen and as boys their age are, a period is a major inconvenience to be ignored or resented. This is the time when we often go on the pill, use tampons and struggle with the worst elements of PMS—the monthly hormones exacerbating teenage issues like acne, body issues, greasy hair and mood swings. This is a time when we neither value nor desire our fertility, and therefore often reject our periods.

Mother

For women wanting to get pregnant but who are struggling, a period often means a failure, the lack of fertility, and with it grief, anger and despair, exacerbating PMS.

For a woman who is breastfeeding the return of her cycles means extra tiredness to her already overused body, a sense of being swamped by a baby when she needs space to bleed. It can also mean the return of the anxiety about fertility, and if and when another baby is desired.

Enchantress

For women who have given birth and/or are reasonably at peace with their family size, many of these issues are gone and the monthly period gives a reminder of the miracle of the bodily cycles which helped to create her children. But it also creates a time of disharmony when she is required to care for children and needs to retreat.

Crone

For an older woman, each missed period gives a reminder that her years of fertility are behind her and that a new stage of life awaits. It may be the first time that her sexuality is totally unfettered by her fertility. But it can also be an unwelcome reminder that she is ageing. The way that she perceives older women and death can impact her experiences profoundly.

There are more post-menopausal women alive today than have ever existed before on our planet. In many cultures the grandmothers are deeply honoured and respected. In the past to reach old age was unusual—to survive early childhood, childbearing, accidents, disease and warfare and reach the age of 60 would be a major achievement and one that few would attain. To have survived that long was a blessing, a sign that wisdom and fate had combined in your favour. To traverse the inner journey of menopause, a death of fertility before physical death, and enter into another life—a life unto oneself, no longer beholden to oneself or community as a life giver, but choosing to support, teach and nurture—was a position of respectability.

Medicated moon time

The most common form of contraception for women is the contraceptive pill. It is considered by many doctors and women to be a panacea—promising easy contraceptive protection with the added bonus of decreased menstrual discomfort and acne. Many women start taking it in their teens and continue for years unquestioningly, happy to not have to really deal with their cycles.

Many women don't realize that when you are on the pill you are actually suppressing menstruation. The contraceptive pill does not give you a natural bleed, it's what is called a breakthrough bleed and is due to chemical withdrawal. It is not a period at all. The pill works by fooling your body into thinking you are pregnant, it thickens cervical fluid making the vagina inhospitable for sperm and also prevents you ovulating. In my experience many women are not told this when being prescribed the pill, so are unaware.

Lorraine Ferrier

I have not taken the contraceptive pill for years. It was only when leading a workshop last summer, that I realised the extent of women on the pill.

I asked the 30 women to stand in a formation according to where they were in their cycles, placing the moon dial mandala in the centre of the room, and briefly explained the four archetypes of the menstrual cycle. What I thought would be a simple task was anything but. Many of the cycling women did not know where they were in their cycles. But the majority of the women aged 16 to 30 were on the pill. 'Where do we come on the moon dial mandala?' they wanted to know. 'What is our archetype?' Good question!

The truth is: I don't quite know. They are in the Virgin part, in the sense that they are pre-motherhood, they are in the Mother section, in that their bodies are being hormonally tricked into thinking they are pregnant. But they are in the Enchantress archetype in terms of libido and mood. The pill is an artificial state of being. And sometimes we forget that. We forget how new it is in human culture, and to our bodies.

I remember that 'not-quite-one-thing-nor-the-other' feeling all too well. Like many girls of my generation and the next I went onto the pill very early on, before I had gotten a real sense of my libido or my cycles.

My moon time in my teens was hard. Not only did I have the mood swings of teenage girlhood and PMS, but my period pains were so bad that I would often faint in the first couple of days of menstruation. I would be writhing in agony, often on bed rest with a hot water bottle and as many pain killers as I could safely take.

I was a high achiever, with full busy days at school. The mentality around periods was that they got you off swimming, but that was it—carry on regardless, they shouldn't have any impact on you. And so I tried to do that for years.

The doctor prescribed me the strong painkiller Ponstan at first, which had little effect. He told me that period pain would get better after I had children, which was, we both agreed, a very long way off. He then placed me on the contraceptive pill. I was 16 and proud to be on the pill. Looking back now that makes me feel angry that there was no other way of helping me to deal with this.

I felt sad, depressed, as though I was floating below the surface of life. I didn't feel like myself on the pill, but because I couldn't point to any definite symptoms, or explain what that really meant, no one would take me seriously. No one told me it was because I was cut off from my own rhythms. No one said that this is quite a normal feeling on the pill.

I took myself off it after a year or so, only to go back on it a year later when I got a serious boyfriend (now husband). But once again I was miserable on it, my libido plummeted—I always joked that the reason it was a good contraceptive was because I never wanted to have sex when I was on it.

I tried a few different types, each coming with great promises. . . and longer lists of side effects. I was longing for carefree contraception and the added advantage of postponing my periods on beach holidays. But in the end decided it just wasn't for me. The cons far outweighed the pros. . . in fact it felt like a bit of a con altogether. It was not the magic pill I had been led to believe. I concluded that I must be the one weirdo that it didn't work for. Little did I know.

It wasn't until I read *The Pill: Are you sure it's for you?* by Jane Bennett and Alexandra Pope, which shares the experiences of hundreds of women from around the world, that I realised I was most definitely not alone in experiencing these 'minimal side effects' which my doctors brushed aside as irrelevant or imaginary. In fact, fully one third of users of the new generation of pill stop taking it because of depression. This book and *Sweetening the Pill* by Holly Griggs Spall added hard evidence to my own personal experience of the pill which doctors had ignored, denied or belittled. This has been a consistent and underreported issue since the advent of the pill in the late 1950s. According to Jonathan Eig in his book *The Birth of the Pill*, almost half of initial (co-opted) trial participants quit the first pill trials due to abdominal pain or nausea. In a second trial its creator, 'chose to ignore serious side effects, which he deemed "psychosomatic". It was one of the boldest and most controversial field trials in the history of modern drugs.'

Some of the effects are scary, especially those that are permanent. Your levels of globulin, which binds testosterone and affects the libido, are four times lower, ***forever***, if you have taken the pill. You have a doubled risk of breast and ovarian cancer if you took it under the age of twenty. Ditto brittle bones. All things I wished someone had told me then. These are invisible risks, that deliver serious, life-altering health impacts later in life.

For a thorough round up of the scientific research and personal experiences of women on the pill—from depression to weight gain, loss of libido, infertility, thrombosis—I highly recommend these books, to give you the insight that our doctors should, so that you can make properly informed decisions before making such a major health decision.

Looking back I mourn those lost years of unmedicated girlhood, of my sexuality blossoming unhindered by chemical interference. I am angry about the potential lifelong side effects which went unmentioned. I am sad that I trusted the doctors. And I am very glad that there is now more information out there to help girls and women make properly informed decisions.

Once we were married my husband and I learned the Natural Fertility Awareness method (outlined below). It gave me a huge degree more understanding and awareness of my body and its changes. I remember leaving the clinic totally inspired and saying to my husband: '*why* don't they teach that in schools? Every girl should know that about her body.' It set me off on my mission to inform girls and women about their bodies and fertility.

AND YOU?

Have you ever been on the pill or other hormonal contraceptives?

How was it for you?

Did you have side effects? What were they? Were they taken seriously?

Why did you go onto it? And what made you come off it?

How might you share your knowledge with other girls and women?

FERTILITY AWARENESS

by natural fertility expert Lorraine Ferrier

When we're taught that it's easy to get pregnant (mainly at school) we unconsciously believe we don't need to think about our fertility. This is definitely not the case as in the UK one in seven couples are infertile (one in eight in the US) and there is a 15–20% miscarriage rate. These statistics are not meant to scare you, but to make you aware: there is a powerful difference.

You don't have to be a genius to do the maths and couple this (no pun intended!) with the number of days you are fertile in your cycle to realise the importance of looking after your fertility. Out of your menstrual cycle of roughly 28 days (although let's stress that every woman's is unique) the egg only survives for 18–24 hours and sperm lasts five, sometimes seven days in fertile conditions.

Shifting our perception of our fertile lives from 'preventing pregnancy' to 'preserving fertility' allows us to take charge of our bodies and understand its ebbs and flows way before we even think about getting pregnant. It's important for both our mental and menstrual health.

Charting your fertility

There are many types of charting that you may have heard of such as the Calendar Method, Billings, Creighton or Rhythm Method. I will be sharing the Sympto-Thermal Method of Natural Family

Planning, a 'double check' method which is scientifically proven and approved by the World Health Organisation. The Sympto-Thermal Method uses the fertility indicators of cervical fluid and sensation along with a rise in the basal body temperature to accurately predict fertile phases.

The Sympto-Thermal Method can also be used for pregnancy prevention (contraception) and as such is a valuable life skill.

In this chapter we give an overview of fertility awareness, but to use the Sympto-Thermal Method for contraception reliably you need to learn how to interpret your chart which we don't detail here.

(You can download a Fertility Joy chart at lorraineferrier. com/ resources)

There is a myriad of information online about fertility charting but using a qualified professional is always advantageous especially if you are using the method as a contraceptive. A specialised fertility professional will be able to inform you how your unique lifestyle affects your fertility e.g. how some medications such as cough medicine, natural or otherwise, impact fluid secretions. They will also have a network of trusted fertility experts to refer you to.

Your natural signs and symptoms of fertility

Cervical Fluid

The quality and quantity of cervical fluid, sometimes called vaginal discharge, (the colour, amount and texture) changes throughout your menstrual cycle. At the beginning of your cycle it is thicker and may be scant or white, ensuring that no sperm can enter the cervix (at the top of your vagina). As your cycle continues the fluid becomes more amicable to sperm transport and survival (becoming thinner, copious and may appear stretchy) indicating that ovulation is about to occur.

How To: Each time you go to the toilet, before passing urine, wipe your vulva area and check your cervical fluid on the toilet paper. This is done throughout the day and a summary recorded on your fertility chart. All fluid is noted. Do not check mucus on your underwear as this will give an inaccurate record.

In your own words describe the 'CAT': Colour, Amount and Texture. One description in each category needs to be noted to enable your chart to be interpreted correctly. Below are several examples from each category:

O Colour—clear/white/creamy

O Amount—lots/moderate/little/nothing

O Texture—slippery/stretchy/thick/pasty

It's your chart so use words or a key that you are comfortable with and can understand. Keep it simple.

Note: Fertile-type mucus is watery and stretchy to aid sperm survival but fluid that is not watery may also keep sperm alive. When you begin to chart it's advisable to have sex every other day as sperm can sometimes get muddled with your cervical fluid description.

Sensation

In addition to cervical fluid the sensation at the entrance of the vagina is used as another fertility indicator of this method—you are more fertile at wet times in your cycle i.e. optimum swimming conditions for sperm.

How To: Throughout the day note the feeling at the entrance to your vagina (the vulva area). For example, when you are on your period you will feel noticeably wetter than at other times. Or perhaps you notice when you feel horny that you are wetter—when your libido rises it's due to hormonal fluctuations increasing your fertile fluid.

Summarise your observations at the end of the day: dry, damp, moist, wet or nothing. When you are on your period just leave this section blank.

Cervical Position

Changes in the cervix can also be charted as the position, openness and texture of the cervix changes throughout your menstrual cycle.

Changes in the position of your cervix throughout your cycle also aid in identifying your fertile times. These changes can be felt at the top of your vagina with your fingers. The first change usually occurs four to five days before you ovulate. During the fertile phase your cervix can be higher in the vagina, softer to feel, more open and a little dimple felt at the entrance to the cervix. This is a useful additional check when you are finding it hard to describe your mucus pattern. Some couples find that they can feel the position of the cervix during sexual intercourse at some times during their cycle—when the cervix is lower there may be some discomfort.

How To: Check your cervix around the same time every day, but not immediately upon rising in the morning or after a bowel motion.

If you have ever used tampons or a menstrual cup the method is the same. Insert one or two fingers into your vagina either from standing, a slight squat or with one leg raised on a chair or toilet.

You need to observe the position, feel, opening and tilt of the cervix.

- O Position—is it low/raised/in between?

- O Feel—is it firm (f) (like the tip of your nose)/soft (s) (like your lips)?

- O Opening—is it opened or closed?

○ Tilt— is it back, front or up? You may not be able to differentiate this, do not worry!

Note: The cervix takes months to close properly after vaginal birth and remains slightly open. It's therefore advisable to allow three months before charting your cervix post-partum.

Basal Body Temperature

The basal body temperature (BBT) (temperature at rest) varies during your cycle, rising when ovulation occurs, because of the release of progesterone. It is this continual higher temperature without menstruation that informs that conception has occurred.

How To: Take it first thing in the morning (before any activity) while still in bed—you can't even roll over to kiss your partner! Take it at approximately the same time every day. Put the thermometer into your mouth as far back as possible under your tongue.

Annotate your temperature on your chart, halfway on the horizontal line (to one decimal point). Record the time that you take your temperature within the 'cervix' column if not using, or by the 'dot' itself. Once you have a few temperatures recorded join the dots so it's easy to interpret.

Note: If you are sick or consume alcohol annotate this on your chart as it can affect your readings.

Benefits of fertility charting

If you do start fertility charting you may observe the following benefits:

○ saving time, energy and stress if any fertility issue becomes apparent and you need to be referred onto a specialist as you have a unique cycle record that can be summarised by a qualified professional

○ seeing in real time how alcohol or stress affects your cycle motivating you to make any necessary changes

○ observing if and when you are ovulating (not all women ovulate on day 14 as some medical professionals have you believe. And it is perfectly normal not to ovulate on each cycle, although if this pattern is sustained do seek outside help)

○ allowing you to see your fertile window in real time to pinpoint the best time for conception to occur

○ measuring the length of time it takes from ovulation to menstruation (the luteal phase) this needs to be more than ten days in order to avoid miscarriage if you are pregnancy planning

Many women enjoy learning to chart, especially relearning facts about their reproductive system that they had long forgotten when taught at school. Men particularly enjoy hearing about their partner's cycle as it is a discussion that does not (under normal circumstances) happen. And charting brings an awareness and understanding to hormonal changes and emotions due to PMS, bringing couples closer together.

Lorraine Ferrier is the creator of the Fertility Joy Program— which blends ancient wisdom and scientific know-how to make your baby dreams a reality. If you want to conceive naturally or have had trouble conceiving in the past check out Lorraine's work.

www.lorraineferrier.com

LIVING AND WORKING BY OUR CYCLES

*With the encroachment of the female into the 'male world',
the advancement of women has been mostly intellectual,
empty of the intuitive understanding and creativity which
is the basis of their nature. There are no archetypes or
traditions to guide women on their needs and abilities
in these new modern areas of work and experience. It is
therefore vitally important that women redress this lack,
that they take their awareness of their cyclic nature into
the workplace and general community, help society to see it
as a positive and empowering force on all levels—at work,
in business, in the family, in relationships, in education,
in medicine, and in creating personal growth and goals—
and that they help to build guidelines, approaches and new
traditions for women to follow.*

Miranda Gray, *Red Moon*

Miranda Gray observes in her book *Red Moon* that we live by
solar months consisting of man-made 'working weeks' divided by
regular periods of rest, 'weekends'—whereas a woman's natural
pattern is three weeks on and one week off. If you added together
the weekend-days in a lunar month you would have the five days
needed to rest and reset, rebalance and regroup during your moon
time! It is, as they say, still a man's world.

But things are changing. Awareness of women's cycles is beginning to become more mainstream. Japan legally enshrined the right for menstrual leave in 1947, and Taiwan in 2013 (although admittedly Taiwan's only legislates for an additional three days sick leave a year). In Indonesia women are entitled to two days off a month for menstruality, and in South Korea too. Stop and take that in for a moment! Women get to work around their menstrual cycles. It is a real thing, not just a utopian feminist dream. And it's happening now in some of the most technologically advanced cultures on the planet.

Perhaps the greatest thing I have learnt from researching and writing this book was how to plan my working life around my cycle. I am admittedly self-employed, but with a hectic schedule of contract work, creative work, interviews, teaching engagements and publishing projects, I usually have enough work for three of me. I have to schedule projects around my cycles to ensure that each bit of work gets the best of me.

How does this work in reality? Well, launches and big events are always planned during the mid-part of my cycles (days 5 to 17), preferably at ovulation. And if there is a big event that I am not in control of the timing of, which falls during my period, I ensure that I allow myself extra time, do as much of the preparation beforehand, focus on getting extra sleep the day before, and schedule in downtime afterwards. I am also as compassionate as I can be with myself that I will be more muddle-headed, clumsy, tired and forgetful than usual. But I also know that I will be more intuitive and reflective, which when doing interviews especially, is very powerful.

Because I work mainly with women who are aware of and attuned to their cycles, our cycles are valued as a key part of our skill set and work environment. Together we function in a positive-menstrual environment—asking for extensions or timing changes to fit our cycles, or explaining to collaborators what part of our cycles we are in, so that we can harness the particular energies of the time that we are in. The phrase 'I'll bleed on it' is common parlance, meaning 'let me bring my menstrual intuition and reflectiveness to this, and I'll be back to you in a few days with extra insight.' As a business owner, menstrual awareness and family-friendly working policies are two key ways that I live out my values, and contribute positively to my employees and the world beyond me, by working with, rather than against myself.

Depending on your work and living situation, you will have greater or lesser flexibility to link your work and daily rhythm to your cycle. But wherever we work, we need to practice standing our ground, prioritising our health and well-being, and learning to advocate for ourselves.

If you view the year as a series of repeating cycles, it should be possible to arrange the tasks so that each receives the most appropriate attention and energy at each phase in your cycle.
Miranda Gray, *Red Moon*

You may well not be self-employed. But we all have some degree of power over our days, how we use our energy and scheduling the timing of tasks. We all have some way of ensuring we get time to rest when we are finished work, rather than pushing ourselves to socialise or achieve outside of work during those few days each month.

What is crucial for us all is seeing where our power to affect things lies. Even in the smallest of ways. And then owning that. Learning to voice our needs, or to actively set the rhythm we need can be hugely challenging to many women. I completely understand. You are effecting a one-woman revolution. But know that you, and all around you, will reap the rewards, as you become more productive, creative and healthy. The first, smallest changes, when we feel powerless, are the hardest. But then, once we start recognising the impact of these small changes, we find ways to make larger and larger ones. And in time, as we live these changes, and others see their positive effect, these things ripple out from us.

Going against natural bodily rhythms can create stress... Imagine a doctor telling you to ignore your circadian [daily] rhythm. Ignore the natural inclination to sleep at night, just keep going till you drop. Not only would it be difficult to order society, it would be madness for your wellbeing. But in essence that's what's happening to women when we're told to ignore the rhythm of the menstrual cycle.

Alexandra Pope

Working by the menstrual cycle

Menstruation

During menstruation we tend to be internally focused and our energy is subdued. This is a time to step back as much as possible. Work by yourself where you can. If you have simple repetitive tasks which need doing, now is the time for sedentary activities, ones which do not require too much of your concentration. Do not put yourself under pressure to make big decisions at this time. If you can take a long lunch, or finish early, or take a half day to work on admin from home, then do.

If you can cut back your hours and make them up later in the month, do. Perhaps you can work from home or hire someone to help, or delegate high-energy or decision making tasks, or put them off until later in the week? Cut back as much as you can for three to five days (ideally two days pre-menstrually and for the first three days of your period). And do not take on new projects at this time if you can help it.

This is the time where the right and left hemispheres of your brain are more connected as the membrane between them thins. You will find you have more access to intuitive thought, and will find it comes naturally to reflect on the preceding month, vision the coming month, and find solutions to problems that have been evading you. Use this time to rest, reflect, vision and evaluate.

Be sure to keep your blood sugar levels topped up with regular meals of nourishing food. Stay warm. If you can take a day or two at the start of your menstruation to retreat then do. Later in this book I will share tools for creating your own retreat space. Perhaps you can only manage an hour each evening to yourself—then make that a priority—put it in your diary just as you would with any other important appointment.

Pre-ovulation

Your hormones are starting to increase and you feel open to new things. You will most probably be feeling calm, open, dynamic, clear, energetic and enthusiastic. You will have the capacity for high levels of mental and physical activity. Start by catching up with things that may have slipped during menstruation. This is the time to start projects and new collaborations: organise and prioritise your time and energy to get the best results. Brainstorm for the month ahead, write your to-do lists and tick off all that you achieve.

This is a great time for a clear out as you have lots of energy and little emotional attachment to things—now is the time for spring cleaning. Any fresh starts you need to make in your life: instigating healthy eating or exercise regimes, or searching for a partner, do it now!

Ovulation

Hormones increase your verbal skills, optimising your abilities to communicate and collaborate. You have lots of energy, so confidence and self-esteem should also be high. Now's the time for big events and launches. Give birth to creative projects that you have been gestating.

This is the time to work late as your creative juices and inspiration are flowing—doubly so if it's also full moon. But be careful not to burn out by trying to be superwoman—you will pay for it later in the cycle!

You may feel attuned to other women, especially mothers, and generally receptive to others' input. So seek feedback, schedule important meetings. Now is a great time for team work and collaboration. Now is also the time when you can get pregnant—so be careful, or go for it, depending on your intentions!

Take advantage of your nurturing energy to visit family and friends who you find demanding. Indulge your mothering side with your own children if you have them.

Turn your attention to making your home feel welcoming and full of love. Have friends over or entertain work colleagues. Over the next week or so, fill your freezer and larder with food that you have made to see you through the hungry gap of your late cycle when you will probably not feel like cooking. This nourishing food will make all the difference and will stop you snacking on junk which makes PMS symptoms worse.

Pre-menstrual

Start to cut back on work which requires collaboration or high levels of energy. Do not plan athletic or endurance events for this time. Try to avoid long, tiring journeys, especially across time zones.

This is the time for dealing with frustrations and irritations—

but only if you can allow yourself to interact with a modicum of reason as well as powerful emotion! Do not be too hasty, pick fights or burn your bridges at a whim at this time—it is easily done! Instead take notes on your feelings, tell a friend or partner, allow them to be a sounding board before you take decisive action.

Focus on administration, more sedentary activities, project work which does not require too much concentration or fine motor skills. Allow yourself more sleep and early nights. Avoid evening meetings or late night parties as your moon time approaches and avoid encounters which are liable to make you overly emotional. Now is the time to try more personal creative projects which require intuitive guidance and reflection.

Cycles within cycles

It is important to note that within our monthly (moon influenced) and daily (sun influenced) cycles we also have 'ultradians', meaning cycles which recur regularly many times throughout the day. Dr Ernest Rossi discovered that we have periods of 1½ hours of alertness and focus followed by 20 minutes of required rest or downtime, to ensure optimum functioning. It is vitally important to honour this rhythm throughout your menstrual cycle—on days of both high and low energy. And whilst you may not be able to have a complete break, ensure that you take a couple of minutes to stretch, walk, yawn, go outside, go to the toilet, close your eyes, have a drink or snack at these regular intervals throughout the day—just listen to your body's signals, it will tell you what you need.

HONOURING OUR MOON TIME

Any cycling woman knows the deep yearning for quietude during her flow time. Every ounce of our body and soul calls for rest, while our culture calls us to keep going, no matter what.

DeAnna L'am, menstrual educator

In their book, *The Pill: Are you sure it's for you?* Jane Bennett and Alexandra Pope refer to 'menstruation as meditation' pointing out that it is our own personal Sabbath. Our culture does not honour the Sabbath, a real day of rest, as our ancestors did. Nor do we have dispensation to 'take it easy' during our moon time from the outside world, as the Native Americans and ancient Canaanite women did. And so learning to take time for ourselves and rest is a revolutionary act.

Often when we rest all sorts of uncomfortable feelings can come up (and comments get made). We might feel:

○ lazy

○ like we ought to be doing something

○ that we're wasting time

○ guilty

○ bored

In my own experience creating space for moon time rest and

retreat is vital for my mental health. If I do not, and try to carry on as normal, I get exhausted, physically and mentally. I get resentful and angry. If I am on my feet for most of the day, or doing exercise on the first two days of my cycle I get crampy too, and my flow seems even heavier. I feel literally dragged down. I have found that if I honour my moon time these symptoms alleviate.

Your moon time is the time when you are feeling tiredest, slowest, when your energy is reflective, when your body needs rest, and your mind needs quiet. Creating a retreat space for yourself allows you to honour your body's natural energy cycle.

We all need to create time and space for:

○ retreat

○ self-care

○ rest

○ reflection

Perhaps today allow yourself to sit in stillness for five minutes. Or to go to bed half an hour earlier than usual and drift. Or to write in your journal for five minutes. Just choose one of those things. Then tomorrow, or next month, you can build up to two of them, and so on, until learning to make time for rest comes more naturally to you.

AND YOU?

How do you create mindfulness in your day? Perhaps yoga, tai chi, meditation, a walk, prayer, some journaling time. . .

How might you simplify your life during your moon time?

What little acts feel comforting to you?

In a later chapter I will be sharing how to create a sacred space to share with other women to celebrate your moon time. But before we co-create with (and for) others, we need this practice to be rooted for and in ourselves. We need to learn how to hold space for ourselves, and settle into ourselves. The rest of this chapter will take you through how to create a safe sanctuary, a private moon lodge or red tent just for you.

Often when we think of retreats, we think of disappearing to a beautiful hut high in the hills, or to a silent religious order—or an expensive spa. But learning how to retreat within the confines of our own lives is a vital lesson for us to learn as women.

The most important part of retreat is creating a space apart from everyone, where you will be uninterrupted. Many women refer to it as 'retreating to their cave'—think seclusion, dark, quiet, containment and safety.

In practical terms this means picking both the right time of day, and a place that you can shut a door behind you. I usually use our bedroom, when the younger children were sleeping during the day, and again in the evening as soon as they have gone to bed. (I must point out at this juncture that I have had a baby co-sleeping in my bed for the past six years, so if I retreat in the evening time, it is done with baby in there!)

Or perhaps you can tempt your partner to head out with friends to the bar or cinema so you can use your main living area.

Whichever space you use, be sure to make it feel safe. Ensure that you will not be burst in upon or have demands made upon you or judgements made.

Do what you can,

with what you have,

where you are!

Shut the door, draw the curtains, take the phone off the hook, turn off your computer and commit to not answering the door.

Make your space feel **womb-like, safe and contained**.

Cover up anything which is messy or distracting with a sheet or beautiful throw: the TV, kids' toys, paperwork, general mess. . .

I suggest **gentle lighting**, like that which you might see in any sacred space such as a church or birthing room. Either a single lamp, or candles. This lowering of light levels has a direct impact on brain function and hormone levels. This helps you to shift into a more relaxed, peaceful and intuitive frame of mind and to feel like you have had a real rest.

Perhaps you might like to **burn incense or essential oils**, or massage your hands and feet with a sweet smelling cream. **Scent is a powerful way to set a sacred space.**

Your set up can be as simple or ceremonially intricate as your heart desires.

Make a **hot water bottle**, hot pad, castor oil pack or just wrap yourself in a snuggly blanket to keep you cosy and soothe your aches.

Get yourself a big glass of water or herbal tea. Hold it in your hands and drink mindfully from it. This will help to get you back into your body, and to replace the fluids that you are losing through your menstruation.

Consciously breathe to centre yourself. Allow yourself to settle back into your body, and the whirl of the day to slow to a stop. Allow the two spheres—your inner and outer selves—to come into alignment, otherwise you will be coming from a place of mental chatter, or emotional turmoil. Sit for as long as it takes to allow this to settle.

If it helps you, **do a guided meditation** (perhaps the happy womb visualisation on the Free Resources section of thehappywomb.com).

For mothers or busy working women, these acts alone,

especially the conscious delineation of your own physical space, which you so rarely have, is a powerful tool in taking back your own energy and power. It teaches you, and those you share your life with, about your desire to set limits on others' demands on you during your moon time. Setting out your space is a conscious way of signalling that you need to be alone and that it is sacred and to be respected.

However if you want more to 'do' then I have a wonderful smörgåsbord of activities for you—but, as always, don't try to do them all!

Activities

Journaling

Try journaling whatever comes up in your head: don't plan, rationalise or be too clever. Perhaps write in free verse. I find quite often that the 'voice' which emerges during my moon time is a poetic voice rather than rational linear thought. It speaks directly to me and I sit and transcribe its rich images.

Moon letters

A dear friend and I wrote moon letters over the course of a year. Every moon time we would sit and write a handwritten letter— we shared our dreams, visions for the month ahead, reflections, quotes from books, poems we had written. These were our way into reconnecting with our own cycles, sharing our wisdom and insight, learning to take time out from the demands of being mothers to young children. It deepened our friendship at a time when we both struggled to find the time, space and energy to talk on the phone.

Dream journaling

Our moon time is often a time of powerful archetypal dreams which can stay with us through the day. By keeping a journal we tap into this wisdom, we find messages from a deeper level of consciousness, and begin to be able to interpret the symbols and themes of our own personal dream language. In learning to honour our dreams, we also honour our need to sleep rather than perceive of it as lazy or a waste of time.

Self-care regime

Now is a great time to enjoy nourishing self-care practices—perhaps a face mask or manicure. Take time to brush your hair or moisturise your skin—nurture and care for your physical body.

Meditation/trance/prayer

Meditation needn't be a formal practice. Simply slowing the mind, whilst watching a candle flame, or spiralling steam coming from a cup of tea, gazing at the moon out of the window, listening to the wind whistling or our own heart beats—all of these bring us into a receptive meditative state where we just are, and our mind can let go of control. Meditation is described as listening to the divine whereas prayer is active, talking to the divine. The divine might be your god or goddess, the universe or your highest sense of self.

Creative doodling/imaginative painting/collage

Any creative activities that can be done in a dreamlike state, which do not require deep concentration or planning, but are rather an exploration of colour, materials and mood, are what is called for at moon time. I love zentangles, which are a meditative form of doodling.

Focus on creative work which is expressive and non-productive—this is especially important if you are a working artist—this is not a time to finish your latest commission, but rather a time to mine your unconscious for images.

I have recently discovered SoulCollage by Seena B. Frost, which is a wonderful visual technique for creating your own archetype cards which would be a great moon time project.

Intuitive practices

Tap into your heightened intuitive powers at this time with whatever intuitive practice you feel comfortable with: cards, runes, dowsing. . .

Reading

Now is the time to immerse yourself in a book which feeds your soul—perhaps something spiritual or meaningful to you as a woman. In your menstrual phase you are especially sensitive, so stay away from horror or thrillers which can overload you emotionally.

Whatever you choose to do, take this opportunity to fill yourself full to the brim with love, inspiration, gentleness and beauty.

Daily self-care rituals for moon time

If you do not feel called to create a retreat for yourself, the bare minimum you should do at your moon time is some extra special self-care—this might include:

○ dark coloured underwear

○ pyjamas and clothes that you won't worry about getting stained

○ red towels or dark coloured sheets

○ a heat pad or hot water bottle

○ a manicure/pedicure/facial/massage/hot stone treatment

○ menstrual products that really work for you—perhaps beautiful cloth ones, a moon cup or thick night pads

○ taking time to eat really well

In the next couple of chapters we will explore how to alleviate and heal some of the more uncomfortable and unpleasant aspects of our cycles.

PMS BUSTERS

Our menstrual cycle is our barometer of our being.
Jane Hardwicke Collings, shamanic midwife

PMS (pre-menstrual syndrome) or PMT (pre-menstrual tension) can include any (or all) of the following symptoms:

O abdominal bloating and water retention

O tearfulness

O being snappy, angry, short-tempered, impatient

O cramping

O lower back ache

O dizziness, nausea, fainting

O diarrhoea or constipation

O migraine or headaches

O forgetfulness, brain fog or difficulty making decisions

O spots, greasy skin and hair

O tender, lumpy, larger breasts

For some women these symptoms may start over a week before their period comes and may continue throughout their bleeding time. This is no small matter if two weeks out of every month are filled with physical and emotional suffering. If you are highly sensitive or empathic be aware that the pre-menstrual phase makes you more susceptible to overwhelm.

If you have had a particularly stressful month, have been ill or taking medication, do not be surprised if your menstrual symptoms are much more severe than normal. This is your body using this natural purification part of the cycle to clear itself of the stresses and toxins of the previous month.

In this chapter I share a number of useful natural solutions for PMS. It can take trial and error to find the combination which works best for you. Don't try them all at once!

If you need something more specially tailored for you, then seek out someone who takes you seriously, is well-qualified, experienced and in whom you trust. Many women find that conventional doctors can be very dismissive of PMS symptoms—having the attitude: 'it's just part of being female, so stop complaining!' And many may seek to cure you of your problems by prescribing the pill. I remember that my doctor when I was a teen told me I'd have to learn to live with it and it would get better after I had children—what a great help that was!

If you are tempted to take the pill to alleviate PMS symptoms, or your young daughter has this suggested to her, be sure to read the book *The Pill: Are you sure it's for you?* before doing so, to ensure that you are fully informed about it.

What causes PMS?

Somewhat incredibly, many menstrual researchers have discovered that PMS is a condition almost exclusively found in the Western world. Indeed, it is a complaint that women and medical professionals alike in other cultures have no comprehension of.

Relationships, upbringing, the stress and pressure of living in a masculine, modern world—all these things regularly disconnect us from awareness of our authentic female nature.

Miranda Gray

PMS has been attributed to a combination of: pollution, poor diets, raised stress levels, 24/7 lifestyles and the status of women in our culture. Other researchers put it down to mineral deficiencies—most notably in magnesium and calcium. But again the lack of these, or poor absorption of them can be put down to poor diets, toxins and stress.

In the afterword to *The Wise Wound*, authors Penelope Shuttle and Peter Redgrove state: '*Society apparently has amplified the menstrual taboo by creating a diet [and lifestyle] that is OK for men but which harms women's menstrual cycles.*'

It seems that we have built a culture which optimises PMS, depression and exhaustion, rather than women's health. It is time to start taking this back, one woman's life at a time.

Scientists have described how our physical growth happens at night. New mothers and babies require much higher levels of sleep and rest. And so do menstruating women. For thousands of years farmers have known about the importance of allowing fields to lie fallow to re-balance their nutrients and growing potential.

It is just the same with us women. As life givers we are given the clues in the form of PMS that in order to be healthy, bring forth new life and create new work and nurture others, it is essential that we rest and regenerate.

We live in a culture which demands that we are 'turned on' all the time. Always bright and happy. Always available for intercourse—both sexual and otherwise with people. Psychologist Peter Suedfeld observes that we are all '*chronically stimulated, socially and physically, and are probably operating at a stimulation level higher than that for which our species evolved.'*

It is up to us to value rest and fallow time. We must demand it for ourselves to ensure our health.

The Crazy Woman

The emotional side of PMS is the raw, primal female voice unleashed, your primal power saying 'Enough—I need space, time, freedom and expression—let me out!'

This is the Crazy Woman, another feminine archetype. She was depicted and revered in ancient goddesses: Kali, Medea and Hecate, the face of the goddess of death. But our modern cultures have no place for her and no image of her. The dark goddess is missing from the Western world. We fear her destructiveness inside ourselves and she is deeply threatening to our society.

We dare not admit to her for fear of being deemed 'unable to cope', out of concern that our children might be taken from us or that we might be hospitalized in a mental institution. And so our Crazy Woman side is further denied, pushed away, or medicated with anti-depressants, self-harm, eating disorders or alcohol. Especially when she emerges pre-menstrually.

> *Crazy Woman does not really wish to kill you. She wishes*
> *to maim your talents and paralyse your ability; she wishes*
> *to strip you of all your sacredness. She pulls your sanity and*
> *tests you, trying to pull you away from your centre.*
> **Lynn V Andrews, *Meta Arts* magazine**

The Crazy Woman emerges for me after too much unbroken child-caring time, sleep deprivation or too little creative head space. I get cranky and snappy. If this is compounded over weeks and weeks I suffer from PMS, migraines and depression. The results aren't pretty. I want to see blood, make pain. I want to do damage, destroy everything which on a different day I hold dear. I want to smash plates, slam doors, hurt my children, scream at the top of my lungs, even kill myself. But I don't. So I shout, or drive the car a bit too fast, or stuff my face with unhealthy food. I want to run, to hide, to quit once and for all. I have had enough.

Denial of our creative selves, lack of space and time to be or reflect are lures for the Crazy Woman. She emerges, raging, crying, shouting, threatening, hands shaking, face pale. But rather than let her out, we try to shut her up and then blame everyone else for her enslavement and our feeling of being trapped.

When you are tired and drained and you have given every drop of energy, love, patience. When you need a break, some head space, some body space and just can't get it. Then you feel truly like you are going crazy, like you are dying inside.

And this is right in a way—we are experiencing the psychic suffocation of our creative selves, when we are so subsumed by external demands, when we do not have time to tend our creative fires, to unleash our imaginative power, plumb our depths, to breathe consciously, to reflect, to play.

Honouring your Crazy Woman

How can we find safe expression for the Crazy Woman? How can we be true to her and ourselves? How can we find balance in our lives so that she need not emerge too often or destructively?

As crazy as it might sound, rather than push her away, we need to honour her.

So next time your Crazy Woman comes to visit, don't run and hide from her. Welcome her as an honoured guest.

Copy down her words in your journal and heed them well. Stop what you are doing and drink tea with her. Dance to her wild tune, play your drums with her and shake your rattles. Take her to bed and ravish her with sleep, let her guide you into other realms of your consciousness. Trust her rather than refuse her. Let her lead you by the hand and thank her for her presence.

She is you—your shadow side with lessons to teach you about what you choose to hide away. She calls your deepest soul attention to that which you refuse to shine your light on. She may terrify you, embarrass you, mess up your carefully made plans and your carefully done mascara, but she is your soul sister, your twin self. She has been scorned and rejected, demonised throughout history. Open your arms and your heart to her and her lessons. Welcome your soul sister back.

AND YOU?

What have you learnt about the Crazy Woman—from your mother, grandmother, aunts, teachers, female friends? Was she acceptable or locked away, the mad woman in the attic? Was she papered over with niceness and face powder? Was she medicated with anti-depressants or alcohol? Did she emerge in screaming fits or suicide attempts?

Grab a sheet of paper and put down all the words you associate with her.

Take your journal and write down her last few visits—why did she come? What invited her into your life? How did she express herself? What did she want? What was her message?

Do the creative archetype exercise from earlier, this time focused on The Crazy Woman.

And now that you have a tangible sense of her, how could you represent her or symbolise her? If you have an altar space in your house, put an image or reminder on it of her.

Partners and the menstrual cycle

Part of learning to live in harmony with our menstrual cycles is in educating the people we share our lives with—especially our partners.

Women partnered to women have a natural advantage, as your partner will already have some understanding of the rollercoaster of emotions involved in being a cycling woman.

Women partnered to men need to find a way, when they are feeling loving and communicative, to help share both the biological and spiritual insights of the menstrual cycle (this book might be of interest, I know a few men have read it!) The very basic understanding we need to share is how our energy levels change throughout the cycle. You need to explain that menstrual women need more rest, and then work together to find ways you can have the rest and support you need approaching menstruation and for the first couple of days of your moon time. This is even more important if you also work together. I know a number of couples who plan their business schedules around the female partner's menstrual cycle.

Explaining the fluctuations in your fertility and libido are also key, so that he can take an active part in your contraceptive decisions, and your sex life can be a real, loving reflection of both of your sex drives. Many couples are unaware of the peaks of libido at both ovulation and menstruation, and this knowledge is a wonderful counter-weight to the 'negatives' of pre-menstrual issues.

Sharing openly with your partner about your menstrual cycle and fertility and working together to find ways to honour and support them in your lives is one of the best ways to bring real intimacy, trust, understanding and harmony to your relationship.

Blood and milk—menstruation and motherhood

What strikes me reading through a lot of the material on menstruation is that is seems oddly detached from the fruits of the menstrual cycle: children. In *The Wise Wound*, Penelope Shuttle notes that there is no research done on the impact of a mother's PMS on her children. Yet think what a massive impact this has on them. This is yet another area where we need to learn to break the silence and find new ways of living and mutual support.

I saw my mother struggle badly with PMS. She seemed to have it for two out of every four weeks. She was like a bear, and any tiny thing was an excuse for her to shout and scream and behave (in my eyes) unforgivably. It seemed to me to be a 'get out of jail free card' for her moods and emotions: 'It's not my fault, I've got PMS'.

So we all suffered along with her. She was disempowered by her emotions. And we were disempowered by them too. It felt like the whole house was cowering from her and her bloody (excuse the pun) period!

And so when my time came, and for years afterwards, I tried to hide mine underground, because I didn't want to be like her. I didn't want to make it everyone else's problem. But that is easier said than done. Especially, as I was to discover, when you have young children.

Perhaps children are not part of your plan now, or ever. But most women at some point in their moon life will have to balance the constant energetic requirements of children with their own changing energy cycles.

For me this has been an enormous learning curve, because at just the time when I am really starting to tune into my own rhythms, I have three children making demands of me—needing me to wake in the night to breastfeed or settle them, wanting me to play high energy games when all I want to do is lie on the sofa. I find it deeply challenging being able to feel my body's rhythm and know how best I can meet this, and yet be constantly prevented from doing this because of the needs of my children and their lack of understanding.

Chinese medicine describes how bleeding and lactating both deplete the body, and do not recommend doing both. If you are, then it is vital that you support your system with optimum nutrition, extra rest and perhaps herbs.

In other cultures and other times women would not be left to care for children alone, in isolation. Instead it was the job of the community to care for, feed and educate the young of the tribe, and women would share their mothering and household chores between them.

Bear this in mind during your moon time. Join together with friends, let your children play together as you cook a meal to share. Or exchange childcare so that you can both have a couple of hours to yourself.

OOO

Positively menstrual!

So how can we transform PMS? I have found that this simple four part process works wonders in my own life, especially in combatting martyr mentality:

Step one: Feel/identify your needs

Step two: Claim your needs

Step three: Make it your problem, not everyone else's

Step four: Make your peace—express gratitude and seek forgiveness.

As soon as you model how you can positively meet your needs, you will find those around you following your lead and helping to support this. Whereas if you are attacking them and they are having to be defensive, they are not going to feel very supportive or like giving you anything!

Learn to use your power wisely. Own it!

AND YOU?

What is it that you would really like to say? And to whom?

Create a safe space and allow yourself to speak your truth—without needing to justify or explain, simply hear your voice speaking your full truth. Every last bit of it. Ungag yourself. Free your voice. Give yourself permission to let your feelings be as they are. Speak your truth—and take ownership of it.

- O You can do this by journaling, putting your seething, unexpressed, and seemingly inexpressible, taboo feelings into words is a massive step in healing, letting go and finding clarity for yourself.

- O Even more powerful is speaking out loud. So if nothing else, read aloud what you have written in the privacy of your own room.

- O But more powerful still is to be heard by someone else (usually not the person it is directed at, at this point. The purpose of this is to purge your powerful feelings uncensored.) Ensure absolute confidentiality—perhaps a counsellor or therapist, your women's group, red tent, a close friend or partner.

After this venting and release, after reflection and possible feedback, then you can clarify what, and if, you do want to communicate to the person involved, or what action you need to take. Then you can act with conviction and speak in a way that your message can be heard. At other times, simply allowing yourself to hear and express your truth is all that is needed to find peace and healing and to move forward.

Instant PMS busters

Chances are that if you have PMS right now you feel crappy and don't know where to start. You just want to feel better. Pick three of these and you'll be well on your way to feeling good. Can't choose? Just close your eyes, point to one. Then do it!

○ In my grandmother's words: SIMPLIFY, SIMPLIFY, SIMPLIFY! This is your mantra for a better moon time.

○ Try to turn off screens at least an hour before you go to bed and get to sleep in good time.

○ Relish your dream time. Ernest Hartmann, in *The Biology of Dreaming*, describes how our need for REM sleep increases in the pre-menstrual period and lack of it causes PMS.

○ Ensure you have no major deadlines, launches or big stressful events—either get work done early or renegotiate extra time for yourself so that days 25 to 2 are as clear of pressure as they can be.

○ Cook in advance for yourself and freeze the meals, go out to eat, get invited to others' houses, have your partner take over cooking duties, buy ready meals. . .

○ Limit energetic or extended physical activity—no long hikes or marathons!

○ A short, gentle stroll outside does you the world of good to reconnect with yourself and nature and get the energy moving.

○ Or perhaps a walking meditation.

○ Have you discovered womb yoga? It is a wonderful, gentle form developed especially for women.

- Keep your clothing comfortable—especially if you get bloated or chilly at this time. Wrap up warm!

- Do something to make yourself look and feel beautiful—wear a special necklace, a lovely scent, a pretty scarf. . .

- Make no major decisions. Just don't do it to yourself!

- Take time every day for yourself.

- Create your own personal moon lodge—minimum half an hour devoted retreat and self-care.

- Get as much support as you can for any big projects, especially events outside of your control—work, Christmas, relatives visiting. . .

- Be open with those that you are close to that this is a time where you need to be gentle with yourself.

- Do everything you can to make yourself feel cherished, NOT a patient or a victim—your mental attitude matters hugely.

- Scream into a pillow.

- Take ten conscious breaths.

- Have a girly lunch with a friend.

- Let your hair down, your tears out and your feelings be heard.

- Write in your journal. Use this time to vision.

- Get a punch bag and beat it!

- Have an orgasm—they're great for releasing tensions

in the yoni, and they give you a rush of serotonin and oxytocin to boost your mood.

○ Choose one relationship issue to take action on. Do not try to change your world or those around you just because you are angry and frustrated. Just one clear communication, made in calmness, of a need that you have and how you would like it to be met. Next month you get a chance to voice another.

○ Bathe yourself in the positivity of others if you are feeling dark—uplifting books, films, blogs. . .

○ Listen to something that soothes you—music, an inspirational speaker, birdsong. . .

○ Tend your personal altar or sacred space—add something red, an image of the Crazy Woman or the dark goddess perhaps.

○ Do some receiving from your family: get a full body massage, a shoulder rub, a hug, a meal made for you. . .

○ Snuggle up with a hot water bottle or castor oil pack.

○ Brew up a pot of herbal tea.

○ Go to the health food store and get some supplements for yourself. And then take them!

○ Eat chocolate!

○ Recharge yourself with a pedicure, acupuncture, craniosacral therapy, reiki, chiropractic treatment. . .

○ Start a dream journal—note down everything that comes through from your other layers of consciousness at this time.

○ Get an abdominal massage—Arvigo Technique of Mayan Abdominal Massage is created for women's womb health.

○ Try a womb wrap.

○ Cut out wheat, sugar and animal products.

There is no shame in tears.

There is a need for anger.

Blood will flow.

Speak your truth.

Follow your intuition.

Nurture your body.

But above all. . .

Let yourself rest.

HEALING OUR BODIES

Healing is a journey. It is a path we walk every day, not just in a moment of crisis.

Paula Youmell

We can do all the emotional healing in the world, but if we are not nurturing and nourishing our physical bodies we will never find good health. What we eat can impact our moods, create allergic responses and affect our energy levels. Part of our healing journey is becoming aware of how we respond to different foods at different times in our cycle.

Herbs are part of the traditional wise woman approach to health. Cultures around the world use the healing powers of plants to help support the female system from Chinese herbs (often given alongside acupuncture), to Ayurveda (alongside yoga), Native American and traditional European wise woman herbalism. They have been used to promote fertility, abort unwanted foetuses, support breastfeeding, tone the uterus in preparation for birth and to lighten or induce bleeding.

Herbs tend to be much gentler than pharmaceuticals and work with the body, rather than simply repressing symptoms. They tend to have few, if any, unwanted side effects. However, they are still powerful external forces in the body and we need to have respect for herbs, in just the same way as we do for pharmaceutical medicines.

Herbs can be taken in capsules, teas or tinctures. They can be grown yourself, sourced from a health shop or herbalist.

If you are new to herbs I strongly recommend c⟨ ⟩
herbalist or naturopath to help to focus and suppc
If you have used herbs before, then be sure to
herbal book or knowledgeable health food shop a
of any contraindications for other medication you ⟨…⟩
breastfeeding implications and existing health complaints.

Below is a resource of herbal and nutritional remedies for easing
moon time symptoms, and helping you to work with your cycles.

**Please note I am not a trained herbalist. The list of herbs
below is simply provided as information, not a prescription.
Whilst I have sourced these suggestions from a range of
reliable sources and I have tried many of them myself, I
request that you seek further advice before taking them.**

Herbs

The simplest way to take herbs is either as a herbal tincture in
water or brewing herbs (fresh or dried) together to make tea.

Teas

These can be bought loose or in tea bags or harvested from
your garden:

- Lemon Balm (Melissa)—to soothe and relax.

- Red Raspberry Leaf—tones the uterus and aids nausea.

- Nettle—for iron. Tones the uterus, supports production
  of breast-milk and vitamin K.

- Cramp Bark—for easing cramps!

Motherwort—good for cramping during menstruation and easing labour contractions and after-pains.

○ Chamomile—to soothe, relax and help sleep.

○ Shepherd's Purse—to ease excessively heavy bleeding.

My personal favourites. . .

○ Rose-hip and hibiscus—a vibrant red tea perfect for bleeding time ceremonies, and a good source of vitamin C.

○ Cinnamon, ginger and cardamom for warming and soothing.

○ Lemon verbena and lemon balm to refresh and relax.

In *Thirteen Moons*, a herbalist suggests:

○ a combination of red raspberry, cramp bark, squaw vine and black cohosh for general PMS symptoms.

Neal's Yard recommends:

○ Motherwort, passiflora and skullcap for easing stress.

○ *Agnus castus* and false unicorn for stabilising the hormones.

○ Motherwort, chamomile, cramp bark, passiflora and raspberry to ease period pains.

○ Dandelion and parsley leaves for relieving bloating.

Supplements

Another simple way to take your herbs is in supplement form alongside a multivitamin in the morning.

- O Shatavari—the Queen of Herbs for women. Its name means 'she who has a hundred husbands' in Sanskrit. It is used in Ayurveda to enhance the libido, energise, lighten menstrual bleeding and generally support the female hormonal system.

- O St John's Wort—for low mood and anxiety symptoms. Because of regulations this is becoming increasingly difficult to source in the EU. (Note it is not recommended for people who are bi-polar.)

- O Feverfew—for migraine and headaches (can be eaten fresh in salads and sandwiches).

- O Evening primrose—great for relieving PMS symptoms, taken ten days before bleeding starts—especially effective for easing tender breasts.

- O Maca—a Peruvian root, great for energy boosting, many add it to green smoothies along with spirulina for an instant nutritional hit.

- O Quiet Life—a natural supplement combining passiflora, lettuce, hops and valerian to calm anxiety and help natural sleep.

Flower essences

- O Female Essence—a ready-made blend of flower essences to support the female system.

- O Flower remedies (such as Bach): especially Impatiens (for impatient feelings), Holly (for when you're feeling prickly) and Oak (for strength).

Essential oils

Can be used for burning, massage or in a bath—should always be used diluted in a base oil (e.g. sweet almond oil) if applied direct to the skin:

- ○ Clary Sage—brings clarity to the mind.

- ○ Rose—good for anger.

- ○ Geranium—good for depression and stress.

- ○ Neroli—good for soothing, weepiness and depression.

- ○ Mandarin/Orange—uplifting.

- ○ Juniper—diuretic for bloating and swelling.

- ○ Lavender—calming, good for migraines and restful sleep.

- ○ Chamomile—calming.

Cream

- ○ Natural progesterone cream—made from wild yam is good for PMS, menopause, cramps and migraine. Apply it to the breasts or abdomen daily.

Nutritional healing

Eat well, dear woman. Your body needs to be fed properly to be able to stay healthy. Nourishing your body needs to be one of your main priorities. Be aware of destructive eating patterns which you may have developed—eating instead of expressing, or even feeling, your emotions, or dosing yourself with caffeine rather than resting.

Find which foods work for **your** body. Find your own rhythms for eating—and be aware that these might not be what those around you need, nor what you were brought up with.

Honour your body with every mouthful you take. Find your own levels of enough. Discover your own levels of satisfaction. Depriving ourselves of real nourishment during the rest of the month leads to nutritional deficiencies and intense cravings come moon time.

- Keep hydrated—drink lots of water and herbal tea.

- Water or fresh apple juice with fresh lemon juice, grated garlic and ginger is a powerful tonic to support and cleanse the liver.

- Many women swear by green smoothies to boost energy, especially during moon time. Add a large handful of leafy greens (spinach, kale, lettuce and perhaps some spirulina) to your normal smoothie base of banana and juice, blend and serve.

- Consider taking supplements of B vitamins, especially B6 and B12, iron, zinc and magnesium, especially leading up to menstruation, if you are breastfeeding or if you are vegetarian.

- Zinc relieves cramps. It can be found in dark green vegetables, wild plants, seaweeds and nuts.

- Eat lots of green leafy vegetables and dried fruits for iron to ensure you are not anaemic.

- High protein foods such as meat, dairy, seeds, fish and chocolate contain tryptophan—a mood boosting amino acid.

- The caffeine and sugar in chocolate lift your spirits—but

they can also be migraine-inducing or contribute to mood swings and adrenal fatigue, so watch out!

O Cut back on (or eliminate!) alcohol, sugar, caffeine and processed foods if you find this improves PMS symptoms.

O Many women find that they have added cravings for simple carbohydrates and meat approaching their moon time.

O If you struggle with abdominal cramps, bloating, diarrhoea and excess gas throughout the month try cutting out all wheat for a few days and see if your symptoms improve.

O Some suggest that eating red meat at this time can make your bleeding heavier.

In everything you eat—honour yourself.

In every rest you take—honour yourself.

In how you spend your time—honour yourself.

In the people you spend your time with—honour yourself.

In nourishing your body and soul with love and mindful awareness, you learn to truly honour everyone and everything that your life touches.

Healing hands

Since first writing *Moon Time* I have come across a number of healing modalities which are aimed directly at the womb. I have neither tried these, nor am in anyway affiliated with them, but offer them knowing many women who have experienced first-hand relief from them.

Massage

There are a number of different techniques of abdominal massage that are used to heal and support the reproductive organs, digestive system and emotional health connected to these areas. They work by correcting the position of organs, especially the womb, bowel and bladder, and helping the flow of blood and lymph. They can offer healing in an area where there is little other support including:

- menstrual cramps
- fertility issues
- polycystic ovarian syndrome
- menopausal symptoms
- prolapsed uterus
- scar tissue and adhesions from fibroid tumours, endometriosis, and caesarean delivery
- post-partum healing
- bladder issues
- digestive problems including IBS

The Arvigo Techniques of Mayan Abdominal Therapy, based on traditional Mayan techniques, is the longest established with practitioners around the world. www.arvigotherapy.com

Fertility Massage, abdominal massage and other healing modalities are combined to support fertility and women's well-being. The content of the massage is carefully tailored to where you are in your cycle. Worldwide. www.fertilitymassage.com

Mizan Therapy uses traditional healing techniques, including abdominal massage to address conditions involving reproductive organs, the digestive system and emotional health. (Currently UK based only.) www.mizantherapy.com

Holistic Pelvic Health Care is a form of healing combining internal vaginal massage, easing tension in the pelvic bowl, as well as energy work on the female system. Founded by Tami Lynn Kent, a physical therapist, based in Portland, Oregon (USA) who has trained practitioners around the world in her techniques. www.wildfeminine.com

Other more conventionally known healing modalities you may want to check out include Bowen technique, cranio-sacral therapy, osteopathy, acupuncture and chiropractic.

Womb Healing

Womb healings are offered by Moon Mothers, trained under Miranda Gray. They can help to heal and empower women emotionally, return the menstrual cycle to balance and help menopausal women embrace their new form of femininity.

Miranda also runs a free worldwide Womb Blessing five times a year on the full-moon to help women connect with themselves and the feminine. www.wombblessing.com

Vaginal Steams

The vagina is steamed over a herbal concoction, which is claimed to fight infections in the bladder, kidneys and vagina, regulate the menstrual cycle, ease menstrual cramps, aid infertility, and clear haemorrhoids, among many other health benefits.

When it's more than PMS

Some women reading this might think—'PMS sounds like a breeze. I'm dealing with a whole other level of horrible.'

To you I say, please listen to your body. Please heed your suffering. And go to your doctor. Love your body enough to have someone else help you take the burden. There is no shame in a non-healthy body.

There are many conditions which flare up due to the hormonal changes of the menstrual cycle, including:

○ migraine

○ depression and anxiety

○ auto-immune conditions

If your mood swings take you into the self-harm or suicidal range, please seek help straight away. Your suffering is real, it matters, but the only way to make it better is by having the courage to seek support.

If you are struggling with heavy bleeding, intense pain, or other persistent symptoms in your womb area, you need to contact your doctor for further investigations. Do see someone. And then get a second opinion. All of these issues can have major implications for both your overall well-being but also your long-term fertility.

Endometriosis is a growth of womb lining in abnormal places, such as attached to the ovaries, bowel or bladder. It is an extremely painful condition that can cause infertility. And it's as common as asthma or diabetes, affecting one in ten women of reproductive age. It can share symptoms with other syndromes, such as IBS and so can be difficult to diagnose. Symptoms include:

○ sharp, shooting, stabbing pains and cramping in the abdomen, pelvis and/or rectum

○ pain during sexual intercourse

○ extreme fatigue

○ nausea

- bloating

- diarrhoea and constipation

- excessive bleeding

Polycystic ovary syndrome (PCOS) is a common endocrine system disorder among women of reproductive age. Women with PCOS may have enlarged ovaries that contain small collections of fluid called follicles. Common symptoms of PCOS include:

- obesity

- infrequent or prolonged menstrual periods

- excess hair growth on body and face

- male pattern balding

- acne

Uterine fibroids are non-cancerous growths of the uterus that often appear during the childbearing years. They are also sometimes referred to as leiomyomas or myomas. As many as three out of four women have uterine fibroids sometime during their lives, but most are unaware of them because they often cause no symptoms.

Common symptoms of fibroids include:

- heavy or long menstrual bleeding

- pelvic pressure or pain

- frequent or difficult urination

- constipation

- backache or leg pains

Many women avoid going to the doctor afraid of what might be found. If you have concerns, please go. Take a friend, or your partner. Support yourself in finding ways to best support your health and well-being.

CELEBRATING THE SEASONS OF WOMANHOOD

At her first bleeding a woman meets her power.
During her bleeding years she practices it.
At menopause she becomes it.
Traditional Native American saying

In our culture we have no formal way of celebrating the seasons of our lives as women. Part of my work is in re-instigating and re-imagining the sacred celebrations of womanhood. These important steps on our paths and in our cycles go unmarked, and so we may believe that they do not matter. But they do. And it is up to us to find a way to fully acknowledge and celebrate them. This might be in an informal ceremony alone or a more elaborate celebration with a group of women friends.

Ceremony can be healing. It can set a container in which new visions, forms and identities can be grown.

A ceremony is a formal way of welcoming a new phase and mourning or releasing an old phase. It is a way of making sacred our bodies and their functions, and making meaning of our personal journey, and sharing our human journeys together.

Female rites to celebrate

Here are the key rites of passage that most of us pass through in our lives as women, (note how few are formally celebrated in our culture):

- O menarche (first period)

- O loss of virginity

- O menstruation

- O birthdays

- O marriage or pair-bonding

- O pregnancy

- O miscarriage

- O abortion

- O impending birth (mother blessing)

- O birth

- O closing of the bones after childbirth

- O establishment of breastfeeding

- O re-commencement of menstruation after birth (also after illness or coming off the pill)

- O conscious end of childbearing

- O weaning

- O recovery from a major illness

- O commencement of menopause

- O last bleed

- O retirement

- O death

Which of these do you celebrate already?

Do you feel the lack of not having celebrated any of these in the past?

Which would you like to celebrate in the future?

Are there any of your friends or family who are at an important stage in their lives that you would like to help to celebrate?

How might you do this?

Creating ceremony

We are used to creating ceremonies in our culture... birthdays, Christmas, weddings and funerals. But there are many, many important life passages that go completely unmarked. Part of our re-weaving of women's culture is a claiming of these rites of passage as important and finding ways to mark them which are meaningful to us.

You do not need to be religious, or even spiritual to create and enjoy ceremony. Think of a birthday party—this is one of the most common rituals in our culture—we send out invitations, set a pretty table, make a cake, light candles, blow them out, our friends sing us a song, give us gifts and cards which are meaningful to us, wish us well for the year ahead, perhaps make speeches and then share food with us. A birthday party contains all the elements of the ceremonies I mention in this book.

So even if you are new to ceremony, or a little uncomfortable with the idea, chances are you have celebrated many, big and small, in your lifetime already. And whilst it is easier to follow the well-worn traditional rituals of birthday parties, because we (and our guests) know what is expected, making new celebrations such as menarche, croning or grieving rituals is exciting—as we are creating them fully in our own images—with no expectations.

The most important thing about creating ceremony is not that you follow rules—mine or anyone else's—but that you follow your heart regarding what needs to be said, done, acknowledged. Use the ceremony as a container—a time and space to give words, symbolic gestures, actions and visual expression to your unseen inner realms. A ceremony should be an authentic reflection of, and container for, your unique journey. It should only contain things which support your process, not that make you feel uncomfortable or 'not yourself'. That is not to say they should be 'easy'. They can be daunting and require huge courage—this is to be expected. Rituals are a making real of thresholds in our lives. But they should always be resonant with our values, feelings and beliefs.

Planning a ceremony

Most ceremonies require a little planning and preparation. But some of the best can be spontaneous and instinctive. Trust yourself and the process.

Set a meaningful time and space. It might be on an important day, or a week, or month, or year's anniversary from the special date you are marking. It may held be at home, in your garden, a community centre or in your favourite natural spot.

Ceremonies usually work best if one person, or a small team, takes responsibility for planning and leading them. Get support for the practical elements like setting up and organising activities.

Set your intention for yourself and the ceremony: that it may heal, uplift, support and guide you (and all those that attend) during the process of the ritual itself and in your life afterwards.

Before starting take time to allow yourself and all in attendance to come fully into the moment, and remember the reason why you are there.

Each ceremony should have the same basic outline:

- An opening: a time for participants to centre themselves and connect with the others in the room. Setting the space.

- A celebration of the woman who stands before us, for all that she has been and achieved thus far on her journey.

- A purification and healing of all she would like to release before she embarks on the next part of her journey.

- Making explicit her intentions and new commitments for her path ahead.

- Gifts, blessings, song, dance, words of power, symbolic actions, gestures of love and support.

- A closing.

- And preferably breaking bread (feasting together)—to 'ground' or 'earth' the more spiritual aspects of the ritual in the participants bodies, re-energise them, and bridge the threshold between 'sacred' space and everyday life.

MENARCHE: THE FIRST BLOOD

The reactions of the people close to a girl as she approaches her first period, are carried in her psyche. Whether we celebrate or denigrate her determines the next several years of her life—her adolescent identity. These same circumstances subtly influence all succeeding physical emotional and psychological passages for the rest of her life.

If she is joyously celebrated, she moves into adolescence self-confident and proud of herself as a budding woman. If she is made to feel ashamed of her body, she feels tainted with the shame and self-loathing for being female.

Virginia Beane Rutter, *Celebrating Girls*

In the process of becoming ourselves more fully it is crucial to reclaim our own personal stories and experiences, for in them we will find the seeds of healing.

Now that we have our own language for our bodies, and an understanding of our cycles, let us go deeper in our work, to excavate our lives and find what lies beneath the surface. Let us enter our own stories and reclaim our truth and power from them. The next chapter will offer the framework, and a living example of how to celebrate your entry into womanhood anew—full of love, acceptance and celebration.

My story

The first time I found out about periods was at school. Just before leaving junior school each girl was issued with a little pocket-sized booklet entitled *Personally Yours*. I still remember the cover, a fuzzy anonymous image of a reclining girl with a blonde bob, pink jumper and jeans. We were intrigued. We took them outside at lunch break and three of us girlfriends lay on our backs, legs up to the ceiling in a concrete crawling tunnel in the playing field, and devoured this new information. We were fascinated, not disgusted in any way. I remember thinking many years later that it was cunning marketing. The booklets were compiled by Tampax. Of course they reassured us that we could still swim or ride a horse: just use a tampon! I was reassured. It felt exciting, but calm.

For me it was to be three years before I experienced it for myself. I remember being in my flute lesson. I felt muddle-headed, clumsy, frustrated, and very vulnerable. I cried and cried. My poor, male teacher was as kind and understanding as he could be, and said I was obviously just having a 'bad day'. I went to the toilet after the lesson. And there, to my astonishment was copious red blood on the toilet paper. I felt excited—a sense of knowing that this was a big deal for me, for my life. A shift had happened.

School was over for the day. But it was a boarding school so I would not be seeing my family until the weekend. It felt too momentous to wait or do by phone. I needed to share that I was changed face-to-face. I grabbed my best friend, we went out for a walk in the gardens and I told her. It felt so right to share it with a female friend, and to do it out in nature.

But being in boarding school also had its down sides. I felt a deep shame. I didn't want anyone else to know that I had my period. So I set up elaborate coughing routines when I opened the crinkly sanitary towel wrapper. I spent ages scouring leaks from underwear, and eventually settled on black underwear all the time.

Only trusted friends knew when you were 'on'. We used to watch each other's backs—literally. In the summer term we wore white and blue striped skirts which showed leaks very easily. It was a sisterhood. We had a special code word: 'P', which then, for reasons unknown to me, became 'Mr P'. Then because my father was Mr P, we called our periods 'Stephen', after my dad. What irony to have a male period, though we didn't see that at the time!

My mother cried when I told her. And I told my step-mother too. They were both lovely and so good with any practical questions I had, there was no awkwardness. I swore my step-mother to secrecy—she was, after all, the sisterhood. But at some point, my father figured out that I was menstruating, and was hurt that I had not told him. I got a five page letter from him expressing this. What business is my blood of yours? I wondered. I felt vulnerable for having my privacy, my secrecy, broken, and by a man.

And so it continues to this day. My trusted sisterhood knows about my cycles—it gives them insight into 'where I'm at', my husband understands the intricacies of it too. But with everyone else it feels like a sacred secret, which I don't trust them so much with. For my sisters, they know, they understand, they truly get it, because they've got it too. We have each other's backs.

AND YOU?

Have you told the story of your first time? Perhaps you would like to do it in your journal, at a menarche celebration for yourself, on your blog, to your daughter, to a close friend, at a women's group, in a red tent? Honour your experience.

What did you wish could have been different? Can you make that right for yourself now?

Celebrating menarche

First of all, it's never too late. Whether you're 19 or 49. If you feel that your entry into womanhood was lacking and that this still has an impact on your attitude towards your moon time or your female body, it is never too late to create a menarche celebration for yourself.

Simple steps for creating your own sacred menarche celebration

○ Invite a circle of women to celebrate with you—your mother, sisters, friends, daughters. . .

○ Decorate the space beautifully—red and white flowers, candles, inspiring pictures, drapes, incense—make it feel special and sacred.

○ Dress in red or white to celebrate bleeding and fertility.

○ Have a special welcome—perhaps walking under branches, or over scattered rose petals. Have your hands and feet washed with rose water and your hair brushed.

○ Sit in a circle with the other women according to where you are in your cycle.

○ Read aloud an empowering women's myth (see *Reaching for the Moon, Red Moon, Thirteen Moons, Women who Run with the Wolves* for resources).

○ Tell stories of your first bleeding, how it felt, what it meant, how it was received.

○ Have your head adorned with red ochre, or your hands or belly painted in henna.

○ Join hands and sing or chant.

○ Each create a red necklace or bracelet which you can wear to remember this day.

○ Light a candle of blessing for yourself.

○ Share food afterwards to ground the energy—you might choose red foods and fruits to symbolise fertility.

If you create your own menarche celebration then you will not only be serving yourself in healing and acceptance, but also the women whom you involve in the planning and celebration. Furthermore it will allow you to develop your vision for how you might celebrate your daughter or other significant girls in your life when their time comes.

By creating your own celebration first there will be no sense of jealousy of your daughter for having what you never had. Instead when her time comes, it will be a pure offering of love for her and an embracing of her, rather than offering her something that you wish for yourself, which, if it is rejected or scorned, will feel doubly hurtful. And in this awareness of her as Virgin and you Mother, you will be able to both stand in your own power, in your own places in the circle.

Celebrating menarche for girls

If you are a mother of daughters you may want to allow the idea of how to celebrate their entry to womanhood to gently percolate for a few years so that when the time comes you are not caught off-guard, unsure of how to respond.

It is important to remember the sense of vulnerability we feel at puberty about our bodies, and the need for privacy. Do not impose a celebration on your daughter. Celebrate her as she is, in a way which makes her feel special and loved, not in the way that you would have wanted, or an intricate ceremony that the books suggest. It might be a special dinner out, or a box of carefully chosen gifts on her pillow. Allow for the fact that although you might want to share your wisdom, she might not want to hear it!

Before embarking on planning a menarche celebration, take some time to reflect—either in thought or by journaling your responses to the following queries:

○ Why do you want to celebrate her menarche?

○ How do you want her to feel about her body, about being a woman?

○ How does she feel about periods?

○ How is your relationship with her at the moment?

○ How would you like it to be?

○ How was your relationship with your mother at her age?

○ How is it now?

○ Are you at peace with your own menarche? If not, what do you need for yourself firstly?

○ Has she ever experienced—either first-hand, or through hearing you talk—any sacred feminine ceremonies? If she or you both are beginners to this, be very mindful of your comfort zones.

Before planning anything, be sure to **clarify your intention**— everything you plan should have the express and implicit intention of making her feel:

○ appreciated

○ included

○ loved

○ accepted

○ special

○ grown up

○ welcomed into your circle of women

We often try to keep our precious babies as little girls. Use her menarche celebration to show that she is growing into a woman and that you honour and respect that.

If she has a godmother or aunt who is close, why not involve her in the planning? If she doesn't this might be a good opportunity to appoint a godmother/moon mother/mentor/auntie. This woman (perhaps a friend of yours, or a mother of one of her friends) is asked to act as her official friend and mentor through her teen years when she may not feel able to approach you, but needs the advice of an older woman whom she (and you) respects and trusts. We all need many mothers in our lifetimes—let her know that this is OK with you.

This is also a good time to tell her about fertility, her cycles and perhaps more about sex, if you haven't already, or deepen her more basic knowledge. Help her to connect what objective knowledge she has about fertility to her own body. Share with her the reality of her own potential to nurture life, and with it the responsibilities. This must of course be guided very much by her own level of maturity and your family's beliefs: a girl reaching her menarche at nine is at a very different place in her personal and sexual development to one who is fourteen.

You might also choose to celebrate with an intimate circle of friends and family. Or to share the celebration with other girls of the same age. Perhaps you would both feel more at ease with a one-to-one celebration. You might choose to involve others in this by asking your close friends and family to send her gifts, letters and cards which you can present her with in private when her day of bleeding comes. Judge it according to her feelings of sociability and comfort in groups or with intimacy.

Activities to celebrate your daughter's menarche

This is a list of possible activities—you do not need to try to do them all!

- ○ write her a letter
- ○ get her ears pierced
- ○ let her choose a daring new haircut
- ○ give her a moon journal
- ○ take her out to dinner
- ○ have a special dinner at home
- ○ give her flowers
- ○ make a cake
- ○ buy her her own red towels
- ○ make or buy her her own pouch for sanitary towels
- ○ give her her first handbag
- ○ or a beautiful piece of jewellery to mark the occasion
- ○ make her up with lipstick, Kohl and bright nail polish
- ○ put together a box of goodies—perhaps a copy of *Reaching for the Moon*, a journal and nice pens, some washable pads, a card with some words of love and a special piece of jewellery. Some mothers put a

box of gifts together over a few years, as they come across special items, and to help spread the cost, and the pressure.

All of these activities seek to welcome your girl into the world of women, doing and sharing 'grown up' activities with her as a means of loving acceptance into the next stage of her life's journey.

As her mother you might want to share with her your memories of:

○ your first period

○ being a teenager

○ your pregnancy with her and her birth (or adoption)

You might also want to vocalise:

○ your hopes and wishes for her in her life

○ an acknowledgement of her growing beauty, power and spirit

○ a conscious letting go of her as your little girl and an embracing of her as a young woman forging her own life

All of this is a part of passing on narratives to the next generation, passing forward their own stories, which we have acted as story-keepers for until this point. And of course, it is another breaking of the female silence.

All our children

Also crucially important at this time is for mothers of boys to find a way to gently and lovingly educate their sons into the mysteries of a woman's body and her cycles, to give him an accurate and respectful understanding of female fertility which he will take out into the world with him.

It is vital that we talk with other mothers about preparing our sons and daughters for adulthood. It is not just 'your problem'. We are all in the same boat, and all hold part of the answer. So pool your resources, work within your own community to find ways to give meaning, and meaningful information, to all our children who are coming of age.

OOO

Menarche: a journey into womanhood

by Rachael Hertogs

Rites of passage have begun to reappear in our society as we recognise the importance of honouring our young people and guiding them gently into adulthood. Ceremonies, vision quests, men's and women's lodges, rite of passage courses, festivals and camps are becoming more and more popular.

I have been working with women and their daughters for many years supporting them in celebrating their rite of passage.

The first period is known as *menarche*. Tribal traditions have celebrated menarche for thousands of years. Some rituals include the whole tribe, others are more private, shared amongst close women friends and family. Some are quite extreme, including genital mutilation, cutting, scarring and tattooing, whilst others are more gentle—being fed, massaged and sung to.

I believe how a young woman is guided through this experience can affect her for the rest of her life.

A modern menarche celebration

I have been taking part in the menarche ceremony preparation at Sacred Arts Camp for a number of years—running workshops with the young women and their mothers, teaching them about charting their cycle, making moon necklaces, decorating red and white candles. . .

What I love about this ceremony is that it is open to any woman who hadn't been celebrated at her menarche, as well as all the girls who have recently begun to bleed. So the ages of those taking part can be from ten to forty! It also involves the men, the grandmothers, the very young girls—anyone who wants to join in can have a role.

All week women meet in my moon lodge tipi to co-create the ceremony—deciding what songs will be sung, what dances to dance, finding musicians, collecting red and white clothes for the women taking part, choosing who will take which role. . .

Meanwhile the young women choose a Moon Mother who will attend the ceremony with them holding their hand and reassuring them, bringing them a gift, helping them to get ready. They might share blood stories with them and as part of the ceremony they dream them a 'moon name' the night before the ritual.

Many Moon Mother/Moon Daughter relationships continue years after the ceremony—even though girls may choose a woman who they only see once a year at camp! They also choose a Moon Father—someone older who can be another 'wise father figure' in their life and who will also make them a crown of leaves and flowers for the ceremony. The Moon Fathers have a powerful role in the ritual, bringing in the male energy.

Other men of the community get involved too. They meet to prepare—perhaps creating a song for the ceremony, as well as sharing stories with each other about men's traditions and honouring women. Their part in the ceremony is to 'guard' the sacred ceremonial space by dressing as 'warriors' and walking around the outside perimeter whilst drumming and chanting.

The ceremony

Each year the ceremony is slightly different. The ritual begins with the decorating of the space. Our big top is draped with whatever cloths and sheets we have, flowers are placed in vases and jars, an entrance is made from willow and flowers. We light candles and incense and raise the energy by singing and chanting while we decorate and smudge ourselves with white sage.

All the women dress up: white if they haven't begun to bleed yet, red if they're a bleeding woman and black/purple for the menopausal women.

While this is happening the young women get ready with their Moon Mothers in the moon lodge, being anointed with sacred water and dressing in white, with a white ribbon in their hair.

Walking in to a big top filled with over 200 women singing is a powerful experience! They sing and dance for the girls and their Moon Mothers, and then leave to change the girls from white to red. As each one leaves the space, they turn and call out their name symbolizing leaving the 'girl-child' part of themselves behind.

While we help them change in the moon lodge, the ceremony continues with the passing of the 'yoni cushion' as a talking stick. As it is passed, each woman who holds it speaks three words to summarise their bleeding experience, words like: connected, pain, loss, renewal and even 'I'm not pregnant!'

After that songs and chants are shared until the young women re-enter, dressed in beautiful red clothes. The singing continues in honour of them and then there is the ceremonial hair cutting— once again symbolising the letting go of their childhood. The hair with the white ribbon is cut away and they are anointed with a red ochre crescent moon on their forehead, to remind them of their moon connection and the rhythm and flow of the moon. They drink from the sacred goblet (blackcurrant juice!) and the Moon Mothers step forward to bless them with gifts and their new 'moon names' are whispered to them.

Now is the time for the men to enter! The Grandmothers have been guarding the entrance the whole time and now step back to allow the men in. But first they are challenged: 'Do you come in to this space with love and respect for your sisters?' To which of course they answer yes!

The Moon Fathers step forward and crown their Moon Daughters, as the rest of the men sing their song. In return, our gift to the men for protecting our space is to share with them a blood mystery story, told by one of our amazing storytellers. After that the musicians play, joined by the drummers and it is time to celebrate and dance the evening away!

The young women leave with their Moon Mums to go back to the moon lodge for chocolate cake and to ground themselves after the ritual. Later that night we have a women's sweat lodge— the perfect ending to a wonderful day!

Reprinted with the author's permission. A longer version of this article first appeared in *Juno* magazine in 2010.

Rachael runs a UK based website, Moontimes, which sells cloth menstrual pads, books and a whole host of products related to menstruation. She is the author of *Menarche—a Journey into Womanhood* which includes articles and stories about menarche, ideas for celebrations, tips for connecting to and charting your cycle, book recommendations, poems and much more. She is also the creatress of the yoni cushion mentioned in the ritual—see her website for photos!

www.moontimes.co.uk

www.rachaelhertogs.co.uk

www.sacredartscamp.org

MENSTRUAL CEREMONIES

They say that salt water is the cure for everything—be it tears, a swim in the ocean, a walk on the beach... or even a salt water gargle. Water is the representative element for women— fluid, ever-changing, sometimes calm and reflective, sometimes turbulent and dangerous. If you are feeling unsettled, water is often the most balancing element to restore you to yourself. Just as the moon most strongly influences our flows, so it influences all water on the planet—the tides and even the water uptake of plants.

Water can be used therapeutically in many different ways:

○ we can take it in through our senses—a walk on the beach or by a river

○ sitting by a waterfall or garden water feature

○ immersion by swimming, showering or sacred bathing

○ imbibing it—through drinking tea, soup, an ice pop or just a big glass of water

○ steam—through inhalation, in a sauna or simply for contemplation

Below I share with you two ways of transforming the simple acts of tea drinking and bathing into sacred and mindful practices, which bring calm and relaxation to your day and give you a little breathing space, even in the busiest of lives. Both are wonderfully simple self-care ceremonies to do in your pre-menstrual and menstrual phases.

Tea ceremony

As a busy woman ordinary days can often spiral out of control making you feel exhausted and frazzled. Around your moon time this can be totally overwhelming.

Many people drink tea as a refreshment, and for many their tea times are a way of getting through the day—the combination of caffeine, liquid and a much needed break revives them. My mother is one of life's tea drinkers; I, however, am not. I came to tea drinking late in life and still I don't enjoy a traditional cuppa with milk and sugar. It was my time in Japan that brought home to me the ceremonial aspects of tea drinking, whilst the wise woman tradition established the healing reasons for taking time to drink herbal tea.

So if you have a full day and really can't offload any tasks, then the tea ceremony is a centring, healing way of taking time out within a normal day, helping to recharge you mentally and physically.

How to do it

○ Firstly, give yourself permission to take 10–15 minutes for yourself. The tea ceremony can be done with others, but the temptation is to chat and the calming, soothing energy is dissipated.

○ If you can expose yourself to a natural element whilst doing the tea ceremony, the healing, calming effect will be magnified. If it is a fine day then sit outside. Or if you have a conservatory or some indoor plants in your office, sit there and absorb the earth energy. If it is a blustery day like today as I'm writing this, sit by an open fire and absorb the fire energy.

○ Turn off your phone and do your best to ensure that you will not be interrupted.

○ From the moment you turn on the tap to fill the kettle, or enter the café, imagine you are drawing a comforting bubble around yourself. Nothing, bar an emergency will enter this and disturb you.

○ Still your mind as the kettle boils. Close your eyes and take a few deep, aware breaths. Choose your cup and tea according to your intuition—what do you need right now? Perhaps a pretty cup to lift your feminine spirits, or a handmade earthenware mug that feels solid and comforting. What tea do you need? (See the chapter on Herbal Healing for a selection of nourishing women's teas.)

○ Pour the water over the herbs or tea bag and as you leave it to steep, watch the steam spiralling upwards. Allow your thoughts and spirit to soar upwards with it, light, free and unbounded. Breathe consciously and deeply and allow your body to settle and rest. Check in with each part of your body from your toes to your head and release any tension.

○ When your tea is ready, cradle the cup in your hands, feel the warmth. Inhale the aroma of the tea deeply. Then mindfully take your first sip. Allow yourself to savour the taste, to really experience all the sensations of flavour, warmth, moisture, as they enter your body and infuse you. With each mindful sip allow your tiredness to seep away and a sense of calm energy fill you.

○ Take a few moments before you are finished to bring to mind something you are grateful for. I always finish my tea ceremony by being grateful for the water which makes my tea, the herbs which grew in the earth, the healing herbal knowledge of people and the time to reconnect with myself.

○ Take your mindfulness, your calm, your soothed body gently back into your day.

Sacred bathing

Cultures around the world have used sacred bathing as a means of purification after menstruation—from Orthodox Jews to the Japanese. Using candles, heady essential oils or cascades of bubbles, relaxing music and a big fluffy towel transforms a normal hygiene routine into a ritual fit for Cleopatra. I was reawakened to sacred bathing recently by Shonagh Home's *Ix Chel Mysteries: 7 Teachings from the Mayan Sacred Feminine.*

I don't like to take baths during my moon time. I have showers and then a sacred, purifying bath when my bleeding has finished. This is another form of steam meditation and water therapy, and one which I look forward to every month.

How to do it

○ Firstly, give yourself permission to take half an hour for yourself.

○ Turn off your phone. If you have children, make sure they are being cared for so that you do not need to be distracted. Occasionally I have managed to do this with toddlers in tow—in which case set them up with an activity—perhaps filling cups in the sink or stacking blocks on the floor where you can see them. Close the door so you know they are safely contained in the bathroom.

○ From the moment you turn on the tap imagine you are drawing a comforting bubble around yourself. Nothing, bar an emergency, will enter this space and disturb you.

○ Still your mind as the bath runs. Close your eyes and take a few deep, aware breaths. What scents do you need? Do you want bubbles or oils? (Be aware that the two do not work together!) Perhaps strew some flower petals on the water.

- Clary sage—brings clarity to the mind.

- Lavender—calming.

- Rose—good for anger.

- Geranium—calming.

- Neroli—soothing, good for weepiness or depression.

- Mandarin/orange—uplifting.

- Juniper—diuretic for bloating and swelling.

- Chamomile—calming.

- Add a scoop of Epsom salts to your bath for a real detox and mineral hit.

○ Make it as hot as you can and as deep as you can. This is a bath for luxuriating in. Be grateful that you have the water and fuel to be able to do this, hold in mind other women in the world who do not and send some love and blessings their way.

○ Light some candles and dim or turn off the lights.

○ Choose some relaxing music, an empowering teacher's CD, an audio of a guided meditation. Or maybe just precious silence.

○ Leave your fluffy towel, bath robe, clean clothes or pyjamas warming on a nearby heater. And have some slippers there too!

○ As you take off your clothes imagine you are taking off the suffering of the day. Look with love at your body. Stroke it gently, with great love and appreciation.

○ Ease yourself gently into the bath. Lie back, take a deep breath into your belly, and exhale deeply, imagining all the stress of the day leaving your body as you do. Close your eyes and take a few more deep breaths. Feel yourself safe, warm and relaxed, contained within a loving, nurturing womb.

○ After a while, open your eyes and adjust to the dim light. Allow yourself to really experience all the sensations of scent, warmth, moisture, as they surround your body and infuse you.

○ Watch the steam spiralling upwards. Allow your thoughts and spirit to soar upwards with it, light, free and unbounded. Breathe consciously and deeply and allow your body to settle and rest. Check in with each part of your body from your toes to your head and consciously release any tension.

○ Gently and lovingly wash yourself from top to toe with a special loofah or sponge and some indulgent shower gel or exfoliant. Be appreciative of each and every part of your body as you wash it. Focus on the beauty and functionality of each part.

○ Take your time emerging from the bath so as not to be light headed. Dry yourself with loving care and attention. Moisturise or oil your skin and brush your hair.

○ Take your mindfulness, your calm, your soothed body gently back into your day, being sure not to catch cold.

MOURNING MOON

Freeing the body inevitably leads to freeing the heart. Emotions need to flow like the blood circulating in the body. When our emotional arteries are blocked, when our heart is jammed up, our whole life lacks vitality.

Gabrielle Roth

It's all very well to talk about welcoming your moon time. But what if the splash of red is the last thing you wanted to see?

○ Perhaps you are trying, and struggling, to get pregnant, and the appearance of your period feels like confirmation of another failure.

○ Maybe your period means another round of expensive and exhausting IVF has failed.

○ Or you are a few days late. . . or weeks. . . and you have mixed feelings about it.

○ Perhaps you are hoping that you are pregnant, or know that you are. This is not just a period, this is a miscarriage, and with it might come heartbreak, soul wrenching loss.

○ Or it is a reminder of an abortion—wanted or unwanted?

○ Maybe with moon time comes a lot of pain and
   suffering because of health complications.

It is more important than ever at these times to follow the
private moon lodge/self-care process.

Techniques for dealing with loss

When we are suffering, physically or emotionally, our first
reaction is usually to avoid or numb the pain. It is a basic instinct,
rooted in our desire to be free of suffering.

What I have learned, time and again, is that this is only a
temporary solution. The more we ignore it, the deeper it goes.
The first step in healing physically or emotionally, is to feel our
pain. To be there with it. I don't say this lightly: *it is one of the
hardest things in the world.* And often something that we cannot
do alone. The first thing we need to be able to move into, and
eventually through, our pain, is safety. A held space, loving arms,
an accepting listener. It may be a loved one, or a professional, but
pets and even trees and places alone in nature can provide this
'holding' that we need to be able to release what we are holding
on to.

Moon time is a natural time of loss, and the emotional flow
often brings unhealed trauma to the surface. Can you ride its
wave, allow its dark energy to take your sadness and pain in its
flow? Allow your body to scream out its sadness and frustration?
How can you safely let your feelings out, see them on the page,
hear them out loud for what they are, let yourself be witnessed
and heard? How can you witness your own pain? Allow yourself
time and space to grieve, to mourn, to wail. It is normal and
natural and OK.

Some techniques that might help include:

○ journaling your feelings

- making them into art—purge the images, feelings, words out of you creatively—pour out your pain, uncensored and raw

- speaking with someone you trust—perhaps in person with a special friend, sister or mother

- writing an email, letter or blog post

- phoning a support line, speaking to a trained, empathic stranger in complete confidentiality

- talking to your healthcare practitioner or counsellor, or finding one you can build a trusted relationship with

- beating a pillow, or lying on your bed and thrashing your arms and legs

- singing, stamping, wailing, dancing, screaming— moving and vocalising however you can

- dissolving into the sadness

- allowing yourself to be held, to be rocked and cradled like a baby and comforted

- allowing someone to brush your hair, to stroke your hand, to rub your shoulders. Feeling that love and care and expecting nothing more from yourself than to be a conduit of your feelings.

- booking yourself a massage or bodywork, or allowing someone to gift this to you

- taking time to do a healing meditation or mindfulness practice

- wearing a flower for remembrance

- keeping mementos—photographs, drawings, a symbol, a piece of clothing, a physical reminder—close to you, in a locket, your handbag or on your dressing table, a private shelf or drawer

O   having a place in nature—the ocean, a special tree, a mountain—to go to when you feel bereft

O   picking or buying yourself some flowers, making a garland or wreath

O   holding a ceremony or ritual—either by yourself or with your partner, a close circle of friends or your support group

A ceremony for loss

Set a meaningful time and space. It might be a week, or month, or year's anniversary from the date of your loss. It may be at home, in your garden, at the place the loss happened, in your favourite natural spot. No loss is too small, too insignificant. No date is too soon or too late.

Set your intention for yourself and the ceremony, that it may heal, uplift, support and guide you during the process of the ritual itself and in your life afterwards.

Take time to bring yourself into the moment, and remember the reason why you are there. Bring to mind the loss that you are mourning and hold it tenderly in your heart. Have an object with you to remember your loss—perhaps a photograph or piece of clothing you associate with the event.

Be aware of where in the process of grieving you are—are you angry, sad, or simply needing to remember and pay respects? The activities you choose to do in the ceremony will vary according to your emotional state—if you have a lot of pain or anger, then drumming, ripping, tearing and movement might be what you need to release the intensity. If it is more sadness, then words or images might be all you need to allow your emotions to flow and release so that you can experience healing.

- O You may want to sing, chant, drum, scream, yell.

- O Bury or burn something in the ground to represent your loss—perhaps a clay figurine, a journal page, a drawing full of pain. Watch the smoke rise and float off. Feel the earth on your hands.

- O Rip a piece of fabric or paper to symbolise your hurt and feeling of being torn apart. Tear paper into tiny pieces and throw the pieces to the wind.

- O Pause. Allow the feeling of release, the feeling of connection to the earth, to the processes of life going on all around you. Notice that your clay or paper or the smoke is already in the process of transforming into a new form: new soil or air that in turn supports new life.

- O Do something that speaks of new life—plant a tree or seed.

- O Read aloud a blessing, prayer, inspiring piece of writing or invocation.

- O Speak aloud your hopes and dreams and vision of the future.

- O Finish with a song or a favourite piece of music which fills you with hope and joy.

- O Ground your energy by holding hands, eating and drinking and resting.

It is real. It is allowed. It is enormous.

It is not the end of everything.

Even though it might feel like it.

You will never forget.

But you can heal, you will heal.

If your loss was a while ago, do not be surprised if these feeling re-emerge every moon time. Take the opportunity each time to work through them more deeply, to heal yourself a little more, so that you might free yourself from being bound to them.

Allow that as your blood flows, your tears flow too. Allow yourself to empty, to shed a skin, to feel the darkness and be in that place. Allow the release. Trust the emptiness. The liminal. The in-between space of not knowing. Honour yourself deeply in your numbness, your pain, your fear, your anger.

And then, as your body begins its journey to ripeness and fertility once more, allow yourself to follow your body's lead back into the light, embracing life in its fullness and renewed possibilities.

RED TENTS AND MOON LODGES

At best, the Red Tent Temple times are like homecomings for us.

**ALisa Starkweather, foundress of the
Red Tent Temple Movement**

Red tents are a place where women are allowed to Be *rather than continually* Do.

DeAnna L'am, menstrual educator

Around the world a new consciousness is springing up, a yearning to honour our female experience, to make spaces and communities that support and nourish us as women, and to create new rituals to replace those long ago lost.

The red tent is one such idea that resonates strongly with many women. In sharing the concept of red tents and moon lodges, I hope to inspire you to create your own. With that in mind I want to share with you a variety of voices from around the world—brave souls who are visioning a more beautiful, creative, empowered way of being a woman.

What is a red tent?

The idea of the red tent was introduced by Anita Diamant in her book *The Red Tent*, published in 1997. She brings to life a group of central female figures in the Bible whose lives were glossed over by male Old Testament authors. She re-imagines the old Canaanite ways in the time of Abraham, where women who were menstruating or about to give birth were secluded for a few days in a red tent. There they would bleed onto the earth and be relieved of all domestic responsibilities. This was where they shared their wisdom, cared for themselves and each other and initiated girls into the rites of womanhood.

Red tents today tend to have no religious or spiritual affiliation, and bring together women from all belief systems and none. Nor are they places where you go for several days to bleed, but rather are a monthly women's space, held for retreat and community.

A **moon lodge** or **bleeding lodge** is a similar idea, but comes from the Native American tradition. It is a place that a woman goes to descend into her depths during her moon time, to be still and experience the magic available to her at this time.

When women started to bleed, they left their homes and families to go to the sacred introspective space of the Bleeding Lodge. The Lodge was honoured and respected by the entire community, for the dreams and visions of the bleeding women brought vital survival information such as planting and healing knowledge and guidance on community relations. When there were questions that needed to be answered, the women would go to the Lodge and ask the Ancestors. All questions were always answered by the Ancient Ancestors. The entire community benefited through the powerful gifts of the women's bleeding cycle.

Since our Ancient Grandmothers probably all bled together, many women shared the Womb Lodge at one time. Ceremonies to honour our womb cycles, celebrate the cycles of the Earth and Moon, and rites of passage were developed by these women from visions and dreams during their bleeding times in the Sacred Lodge. These traditions were passed down in the initiatory rites of the Blood Lodge from mother to daughter.

Songs of Bleeding by Spider

Since ancient times women have gathered together at the dark moon to dream mystical dreams, share wisdom and renew sexual power. Sitting in circle within *The Red Tent*, they are relieved of their daily responsibilities and cared for by other women. All working and doing aside, together they explore the secrets of the cosmos through the gateway of their wombs. They feed their femininity and emerge refreshed, renewed and empowered by what they have shared and witnessed.

In the warm, cosy space of *The Red Tent*, you will be nurtured by ancient restorative practices, giving the body, heart, and mind space to rest in stillness, revitalizing your receptivity to life and love. You'll be enchanted by stories, old and new, of Woman and her mysteries. You'll be fed warm soups, vibrant greens, teas: you will be loved from the inside out. You will have the space, the time, the encouragement to simply Be.

Dawn Cartwright,
www.chandrabindutantrainstitute.com

The dark moon phase, three days a month when we cannot see the moon in our night's sky, was once considered a blessing. In traditional Native American culture, women gathered together in moon lodges. . . to rest, meditate, heal, let go of the unwanted and celebrate womanhood. They were considered very powerful and they were expected to *vision for the whole tribe, helping the Elders with decision making and foresight into the future.*

Jane Anderson,
www.moonandearthconnections.com

Though they are often spoken about interchangeably, it is my understanding that there is a vital difference between a moon lodge and a red tent.

A **moon lodge** is one which honours and allows introspective practices: dreaming, prayer, trance work, visioning and journaling. It can be undertaken with women together, but is often done alone.

Moon lodges have been in continual use within the Native American tradition for generations, and use distinctive Native American language, myths and an austere physical framework. They have been introduced to women in America and beyond in recent years by native elders, as well as Susun Weed and her publishing house, Ash Tree.

A **red tent** is a more communal activity and experience usually in ornate surroundings—one which, whilst allowing for rest and introspection, allows a forum for sharing knowledge, creative activities, ceremony and interaction.

These have been seeded and championed around the US by ALisa Starkweather via the Red Tent Temple Movement, and DeAnna L'Am through Red Tents in Every Neighborhood, as well as independently by a number of other visionary women in Europe and Australia.

The herstory of the emergence of red tents is documented in an e-book by ALisa Starkweather and Isadora Leidenfrost, *The Red Tent Movement: A Historical Perspective* as well as in a powerful film documentary, *Things We Don't Talk About: Healing Narratives from the Red Tent.*

My heart, like yours probably, has been aching when I look into my local area, my world, and see such a great need for the sacred. I see an unmet need in our young to have a place they can count on for mentoring, initiation, and coming into their womanhood with other women. I see an unmet need in our lives to connect deeply, rest and take time to simply be. I see an unmet need for our elders where they can gather to be honoured and share their wisdom. [. . .] And I wondered what would happen in our societies of local places if women were to have a place we could count on where we are respected, supported and held. I understood from the work that I do that to empower women of any age means to bring health back into a community. And the Red Tent Temple Movement is a means to support us.

**ALisa Starkweather, at the founding of the
Red Tent Temple Movement**

A red tent. . .

- O *is part of the spiritual practice of menstruation and the living of the wisdom of the cycles.* (Jane Hardwicke Collings)

- O creates a supportive community of women

- O creates a much needed retreat space

- O honours our bodies with time and self-care

- O provides a venue for sharing women's wisdom and celebrating rites of passage

- O creates a woman-centred sacred space within our lives and the world

They are springing up around the world in private homes,

yurts, festival tents, community halls and dedicated purpose-built rooms. Often draped in red, with beautiful embroidery, soft cushions, prayer flags, rugs, quilts and paintings, they seek to create a soft, welcoming womb where women can come and speak, cry, sing and laugh, where women share healing, body work, energy work, nourishing meals and herbal tea.

Some temporary red tents have been created for V-Day celebrations, art installations and educational projects. Others are more structured women's circles which meet monthly. Some are open to all women in the community, others have a closed membership. Some welcome pre-pubescent girls once a year and run menarche celebrations when their girls come of age.

They are generally held on the new moon, as this is the traditional time of women's bleeding. But you do not have to be bleeding to go to one, if your own moon time is on a different cycle, if you are pregnant, do not have periods or a physical womb. They are a space for all who identify as female. The new moon is often a time for sowing the seeds of intentions that we wish to manifest as the moon waxes, so whether or not you are bleeding it is a good time to go.

What happens at a red tent?

All sorts of things can happen at a red tent:

- O talking circles
- O hands-on healing
- O creativity and art
- O silence, meditation and reflection
- O seasonal activities

○ sleep and rest

○ reading and journaling

○ hugging, laughing, crying, holding

○ ceremonies and rituals

○ singing, dancing, chanting, drumming

○ pampering

Some red tents are free-form, and others are more facilitated experiences. How yours is depends on the wishes and needs of your group of women, and the skills and comfort-zone of the women involved. Some women who are new to women's work, or deal with social anxiety find being in a group of women deeply uncomfortable and need a firm structure to support them. Others have a fear of leadership, little experience in group work, or a desire to simply show up and trust the process, so a free-form group works better for them. Or you can alternate, and have a free-form session one month, and a more structured talking circle or facilitated activities the next.

ALisa's words which follow are particularly powerful for me. Our red tent dissolved because of differing judgements over how a red tent 'should' be.

It is very important that we don't shame or hurt one another in the Red Tent Temples by our judgements about what we think 'should' happen. With time, with focus, with learning, with dialogue in our circles, with experience, trust that we are going to find our way.

At the same time we help the situation with an orientation sheet about what this is. It helps to invite them into a quiet space. Soft music, a place to close one's eyes and centre, a welcoming that invites each woman to let go of her nervousness, her work, her need to belong and be accepted, and simply come home to herself wherever she is.

It is okay to ask women as they enter to have some quiet time first before getting involved with talking. Talking happens. In the Red Tent in my home, there is quiet talking, nap taking, sometimes tears and often laughter. If you have a crystal bowl or gentle bells that can be struck every once in a while as a way for the room to go within, quiet for a few moments, you can interrupt the pattern in a gentle way of it becoming louder and louder.

Women are not going to be comfortable at first with the idea of doing nothing. I have had very powerful women friends who are very active come into the Red Tent and look like a cat in water. The look says, 'what am I doing just sitting here? I should be home DOING something.' But that is the point. We are learning the undoing and for that we look like drowned cats momentarily. Soon those same women are stretched out on the pads or receiving energy work or are journaling, sipping tea, and breathing more deeply. It is really a learning experience here.

www.ALisastarkweather.com

Creating a red tent

So you want a red tent for yourself?

Firstly check online, in local health food shops, yoga spaces, holistic centres or your library to see if there is already one near you. Check the Resources section at the end of this book—the groups on Facebook will be able to let you know of any in your area.

If there isn't one you will need to brainstorm—perhaps by yourself, or more fun with a few like-minded women. Taking time to vision together, rather than rushing in to setting one up can alleviate problems at a later stage, if there are major differences of intention, or levels of work that people are prepared to put in. There are many, many ways a red tent can be run, and what can happen in them.

Holistic visioning:

- O Who is it for and why? What is your grandest vision?

- O What do you/don't you want? What is crucial? What is a deal breaker?

- O What is your one over-riding priority? Community? Retreat? Beauty? This will help to steer you when you feel confused and at sea.

- O What do you like from the ideas here?

- O What don't you like/want?

Practical visioning:

- O Where to hold it?

- O What date?

- O What time?

- O How long will the sessions be?

- O What will you use to decorate it? Where will these things come from? Use what you have, borrow, get creative re-fashioning old bits of fabric.

○ Invitation only or posters?

○ Who to invite and do they need to RSVP?

○ What do they bring? Refreshments, cushions. . .

○ Ensure at least two to set up and two to clear up.

○ Any activities for the tent.

○ Any formal leadership structure.

○ Will you have an online group as well or instead? Private Facebook groups are free and easy to set up.

○ Will you charge? If so, how much?

ALisa Starkweather hosts a free monthly telecall to support women wanting to establish a red tent in their neighbourhood. And the Red Tent Network and Red Tent movie websites have lots of useful resources. DeAnna L'Am has held a free Red Tent Teleconference in February for the past two years, and also runs paid tele-classes to support women who are setting them up.

Do seek out images of red tents online to inspire you. Pinterest is a great source of them—check out my Red Tent board for starters pinterest.com/dreamingaloudnt/in-the-red-tent

Decorating a red tent

Most red tent leaders try to recreate the look and feel of a red tent in an internal room. You can do this with:

○ curtains

○ sheets

○ drapes

○ blankets

O   sari fabric

You can get these from:

O   your own cupboards, attics, drawers

O   friends, family and neighbours

O   dye old sheets red

O   buy cheap red sheets from thrift stores, charity shops, retail discounters

O   eBay has a great choice of very affordable sari fabric

Or you can have an **actual tent space**—in a **yurt, tipi or a bell tent** (which are much more affordable than yurts, and quicker to put up, but have the same feel). A cheaper option still, and one which is quick to put up and can be used inside or out, is a gazebo. You can use it as is or with added drapes.

Creating and adorning a space

Equipment you might need includes:

O   cushions, beanbags and futons for sitting on the floor

O   a kettle, cups, teas

O   candles, incense, essential oils, smudge stick

O   a portable self-care kit—lavender eye mask, hot water bottle or barley bag, a couple of favourite oils and base oil, a foot-bath

O   a portable shrine or altar—with images and objects which are meaningful to you and help you to connect with your feeling of sacredness

O a creative bag (journal, pens, paints, old magazines for collage)

Ensuring your red tent is sustainable

I just want to take a moment, if you are excited about starting a red tent of your own, to caution you to make it sustainable—financially and energetically.

A red tent or any women's group is a labour of love—but should be of many women's love, not just one. Do not work yourself to the bone creating a perfect retreat space for others. After all, you are creating it not just for your community—but for you as well! So ensure that you have support or shared responsibility for:

O set up

O clean up

O finances and administration

O refreshments

O hosting

Guidelines for a sustainable red tent

O Do not do it all yourself and wear yourself out. Allow others to help in serving your community, and in serving you!

O Don't worry about making it perfect. Just make it with love, and aim for beauty and it will be wonderful. Consider it a work in progress which will grow with you all, using the skills and energy of all its members—as it sustains you, so you sustain it.

○ Get support and advice from other women who have gone before you—join an online group or take part in the Red Tent Temple calls.

○ Ensure your decorations are quick, or at least pleasurable, to set up!

○ Make sure not to try to cram in too many activities or ideas—remember first and foremost a red tent is a place to be.

○ Be gentle with yourself in its creation. There are many who may sneer or denigrate your sacred project. I have many of these people around me. They do not need to know about it, whilst you still feel tender and vulnerable. If you feel concerned, keep it private and discrete.

○ It is a sacred space, share it with only those who will honour it as such—ensuring the emotional safety of all who enter it. Ensure you have a clear code of conduct for how women should be in this space. Ours was:

● Speak from my 'I'—rather than for others.

● Share openly and honestly, as much or as little as you need.

● Request at the beginning of each session that women let what emerges in the tent, to stay in the tent—no gossiping or sharing other's stories outside the red tent space.

● Everyone is responsible for their own feelings, for asking for what they need and what they bring into the space.

● Everyone is responsible for doing what they can to help the smooth running of the group.

○ Be clear on how new women are invited. Will you put up posters, or simply have it amongst a closed group of friends? If it is in a person's home then the size of room, and people's privacy might demand that it is invitation only and that people RSVP.

○ Agree in advance how misunderstandings and disagreements will be dealt with by the group.

The more sustainable your red tent is, the longer it will be there to support you and your community. It is a precious resource to all involved, but there is much learning that happens in the process of creating, and sustaining, a group.

Creating your own moon lodge

The original moon lodge consisted of a woven hazel branch frame with a cover made of hides, blankets or cloth—a similar type of construction to a sweat lodge. They tend to be much simpler and less ornate than red tent spaces.

I have visions of creating a moon lodge in the tea house where this book was written, and where I was married. It is a beautiful hand-constructed space nestled in the woods with thick plastered walls, a thatched roof, round fire place and panoramic views over the marsh and sea. Being just one room it feels like a safe womb. It smells of sweet cedar and incense. There are lots of big cushions, comfy chairs and warm woollen blankets. In short it spells comfort and retreat for me. But when I can't get there in person, I recreate this feeling in my bedroom at home.

A dear friend is creating a moon lodge in an abandoned woodland hut. She will let other trusted women know of this space, so that they too can retreat to it when they need. Another woman I know has a summer house which is used for this purpose over the warmer months of the year.

Lodges which are used by many women often keep a lodge book where any woman can share her insights, visions or dreams—these may support another woman in her own process, as well as give material for contemplation.

OOO

Most of us do not (yet!) have a moon lodge or red tent space in our neighbourhoods. And for many of us our moon time is private—we have no desire to step outside our front doors or be sociable.

Perhaps setting up a red tent is not for you, or not feasible right now. Perhaps you do not yet have a circle of likeminded women to share in creating one. Perhaps you feel like you do not have the resources. Or perhaps you just need the courage to act on your dreams.

We are the ones we've been waiting for!

OTHER KEY CEREMONIES FOR WOMEN

We have already explored menarche and moon time ceremonies, as well as touching on mourning rituals. Before we close I wanted to share a few more important ceremonies connected to our cycling years which are so often overlooked in our culture. You might choose to celebrate them privately, with a close friend, your red tent or women's group.

Red thread ceremony

For many different ceremonies that I have been fortunate to lead—at women's groups, red tents, and mother blessings—many women's most treasured part is the red thread ceremony. This is a way of symbolically connecting the women in the group, leaving them with a lasting visual reminder of the ceremony. It is usually the last activity of the event, done in the closing circle.

How it works

You will need a ball of red wool (yarn) and a pair of scissors.

All the women stand in a circle. The leader tells the group of the symbolism of the red thread, which is found throughout cultures. In Chinese stories it was said that there is an invisible red thread which binds people who are destined to meet. In women's cultures it is said that the red thread symbolises our shared menstrual blood, which unites and connects all women. We bind ourselves together with the ball of wool to remind ourselves of the web of interconnections that link us all, so that even when we are no longer in the same room, we remember our connectedness.

The leader wraps the end of the wool around her own wrist (in some ceremonies the wool is first tied around the central candle, symbolising our connection to spirit or the centre) and then throws the ball of wool across the circle—perhaps with a word of blessing, or something that she is taking away from being in circle. The next woman wraps it a couple of times around her wrist and throws it to a woman across from her until all the women are bound together by the red thread in sisterhood.

The leader invites everyone to take a step back, to feel the connection between them as the threads tighten: this is the support we all have to call on. She then cuts herself free, leaving herself ample yarn to wrap another couple of times around her wrist and knot into a simple bracelet. She passes the scissors on, each woman snipping her ties. The women are reminded to remember the feeling of sisterhood, centredness and support each time they look down at their red cord band in the coming days.

In a mother blessing ceremony each woman is asked to leave her bracelet on until the safe delivery of the baby, and to send thoughts of love and blessing to the mother when they look down at it.

A return to bleeding

Whether you are welcoming the return of your cycle after child birth, taking the pill, or illness, take time to mark this event and reacquaint yourself with your cycles. You might choose to:

○ take some of your moon blood and pour it on the earth or onto one of your favourite plants

- O   pick or buy yourself some flowers

- O   dedicate your bleeding time to yourself, to all women, to learning more about yourself, your spirit, your fertility each month

- O   make a piece of art or write a poem to mark the event

- O   make yourself a cake or a favourite meal

- O   take yourself out to a café

- O   treat yourself in some other way—get a massage or a pedicure or body work treatment

- O   attend a red tent

Mother blessing

Mother blessings are a great alternative to baby showers for those more mindful of the spiritual and physical journey to motherhood. A mother blessing celebrates, nurtures and supports a mother-to-be in her late pregnancy preparing her emotionally for her impending birth. It is usually a profound experience which closely bonds the mother-to-be and all who participate in it.

Pregnancy and birth are such enormous milestones in any woman's life, but as a culture we tend to barely acknowledge them. Many women find themselves approaching birth feeling unprepared for what to expect, or feeling isolated from the support of mothers, sisters and other women. Mother blessings answer this need and celebrate a woman's rite of passage into motherhood.

Originating in the Navajo Native American tradition of Blessingways, mother blessings have been developed in the US over the past 15 years amongst the alternative community and are gaining popularity in Europe and Australia now.

Organised and led by a friend or celebrant, the pregnant woman's closest female friends and relatives (usually six–twelve women) gather at her home for a simple ceremony some time in her last six weeks of pregnancy. Though spiritual in their outlook, mother blessing ceremonies do not adhere to any particular dogma or creed. Each is unique to the woman it celebrates and is tailored to her particular beliefs and circumstances. Activities might include:

- opening by lighting a candle, saying a short prayer or blessing

- sharing how you know the mother-to-be and what she means to you

- giving gifts: little indulgences for the mother, babysitting vouchers, organising a 'meals-on-wheels' rota for post-birth

- sharing positive birthing stories, poems and readings

- having a guided meditation

- or a ritual for facing fears to do with the birth and mothering

- stringing birthing beads: each woman adds one and shares her own birthing story

- creating a birth vision board of inspiring images and quotes for labour

- creating prayer flags—each with a message of support or power symbol

- pampering the mother—massaging her, brushing and braiding her hair, painting her toe nails

- making a plaster cast of her belly or painting it with henna or face paints

- ○ giving out candles to be lit when labour starts and organising a 'phone tree' to spread the news on the big day
- ○ closing with the red thread ceremony
- ○ ending with a shared feast

Closing the bones

A closing the bones ceremony is inspired by a Mayan tradition where the post-partum mother is anointed, massaged and wrapped in fabric. This process literally helps to 'close' the mother's body physically and energetically, after the opening which has happened on every level in preparation for and during birth itself.

It is a deeply nourishing, nurturing process, which acknowledges the new mother's vulnerability and need for physical and emotional support, at a time where in Western culture she is pretty much abandoned. I wish I had known about them when I was having my babies, as I know they would have helped the healing of my pelvis and lower back, as well as potentially headed off post-natal depression.

The ceremony is led by a trained healer—often a doula, ceremonialist or someone trained in the Arvigo tradition of abdominal massage, and as well as hands-on healing, provides a beautifully held, nurturing space for the mother. Things that might be included are:

- ○ a ritual or ceremony—welcoming and acknowledging the mother
- ○ a vaginal steam bath with flowers and herbs to bring her energy back into her body and finish healing the post-partum womb

- ○ abdominal massage, reiki, cranio-sacral or sound healing

- ○ wrapping of the lower back and pelvic area using a rebozo

- ○ belly binding, which aids the shrinkage and internal repositioning of the uterus and bladder, supporting the pelvis and lower back as they return to their original positioning

The purpose and intention is to allow a woman to heal from the birth, and to support her moving into her motherhood, physically and emotionally free.

Croning ceremony or wise blood rite

For women in our society aging is often portrayed as a negative thing. Croning ceremonies are a wonderful way to celebrate the journey beyond our fertile years and welcome a woman into her wisdom years.

The feelings and physical shifts that emerge at this time are honoured. Ceremonies can range from spontaneous celebrations at birthday parties to pre-planned ceremonial rites of passage. Some ceremonies are personal, others are shared amongst an intimate circle of friends and family, and others are large public rituals at women's gatherings. The ceremony tends to be performed by a woman who has already passed through menopause herself, but can of course be done by and for yourself. Activities can include:

- ○ a story or guided meditation honouring the archetype of the Wise Woman

- ○ symbols of initiation—a shawl, a wreath of flowers or leaves, a henna tattoo, a medicine bag

- songs, drumming, music or poetry celebrating the later years of womanhood

- an altar with photos of female relatives and friends who have empowered you

- a symbolic acting out of the passage into cronehood, perhaps entering through a curtain or tunnel, or removing three veils representing each life stage: Maiden, Mother, Crone

- lighting a purple candle, the colour of wisdom and mature spirituality

- some women choose to adopt a new name at their croning ceremony. It can be one that you keep to yourself, share only among friends, or announce to the world

- an exchange of gifts or blessings

- a celebratory feast

Celebrating women will change the world

However you choose to mark these rites of passage, what is important is that we acknowledge these life transitions first for ourselves, and then for our sisters, daughters, friends and wider communities. It is vital that we find ways of talking about these rites of passage, healing and supporting ourselves and the women that we know as we pass through the archetypes of womanhood, rather than numbing and ignoring them as we have for so long in our culture.

Celebrating ourselves, we learn once again to value each stage of our lives as women, we learn to celebrate and respect the cycles of nature that we are intimately connected to. We see that we are not separate from nature—or each other. This is vital to our physical and emotional health—individual and communal. These small steps of self-care and celebration hold within them profound seeds of healing and change for the world.

If you have ever wondered if you can make a difference, you can. And this is both the simplest and most meaningful and profound difference.

More than anything else, learning to live at ease in your body, to care for it, to create consciously in harmony with the cycles of nature, to nurture the life you bring through you, to heal and support yourself. That is perhaps your greatest power. It all starts with you and your wise body.

And you can do it.

Right now.

AFTERWORD

What a journey this has been for me—and for you too I hope! What learning, what courage and insight we have unearthed on our travels together. What wisdom we have in our bodies and in women's cultures that we can bring into our lives today.

Thank you for your companionship on the journey. I wish you well as you travel onwards.

If you have enjoyed this book do leave a review on Amazon, and consider buying a copy for friends, daughters or sisters.

Please join me at

- O thehappywomb.com

- O Facebook /The Happy Womb

- O Pinterest /dreamingaloudnt/the-happy-womb/
for a whole host of further Womancraft resources.
Blessings to you,
Lucy Pearce,
Cork, Ireland, April 2015.

RESOURCES

Online resources

Charting

www.lorraineferrier.com/resources
For free charting resources and tuition

www.menstruation.com.au/fertility/mychart.html
Blank fertility chart

www.thebillingsovulationmethod.org
Fertility awareness from the original discoverers of The Ovulation Method—free e-books and charts (go to their resources section)

Charting apps

My Moon Time
www.menstruation.com.au/menstrualproducts/hormonalforecaster.html

Sources of moon diaries and charts

www.wemoon.ws

www.earthpathwaysdiary.co.uk

www.moontimes.co.uk

www.herbalmedicinehealing.com

www.moonandearthconnections.com

www.wisewoman.org

www.moontimerising.com

Leading women in the field of menstrual education

www.lucyhpearce.com and www.thehappywomb.com (Lucy H. Pearce)

www.womensquest.org and www.redschool.net (Alexandra Pope)

www.moonsong.com.au (Jane Hardwicke Collings)

www.moontimerising.com (Giuliana Serena)

www.thesassyshe.com (Lisa Lister)

www.janebennett.com

www.laraowen.com

www.rachaelhertogs.co.uk

www.susunweed.com

www.mirandagray.co.uk

www.alisastarkweather.com

www.deannalam.com

Woman honouring websites

www.dreamingaloud.net

www.optimizedwoman.com

www.wombyoga.org

www.cherishthecunt.com

www.holisticmenopause.com

www.fertilitymassage.co.uk

www.chandrabindutantrainstitute.com

www.thefullmooneffectppc.weebly.com

www.crimsonwisdom.com

www.talkbirth.com

www.redwebfoundation.org

www.yoni.com

www.onewoman.com

www.menstruation.com

www.womansoul.co.uk

www.pixiecampbell.com

www.crimsoncampaign.org

www.wellspringswomen.com

www.womboflight.com

www.goddessrising.org

www.redwisdom.co.uk

www.wisewomenredtent.com

www.thefountainoflife.org

www.thesacredwomb.com

www.birthdance.co.uk

www.nurturehealth.info

Red tents and moon lodges

The Red Tent—Anita Diamant

The Red Tent Movement: A Historical Perspective—
Isadora Gabrielle Leidenfrost, PhD and ALisa Starkweather

www.alisastarkweather.com—for detailed insight in to the 'what' and 'how' of red tents. ALisa founded the grassroots Red Tent Temple Movement in 2007.

www.redtenttemplemovement.com—a grassroots movement aiming to bring a red tent to every neighbourhood. They hold a monthly teleconference to support women in getting started.

www.redtentmovie.com

www.sacredmoon.com.au

www.theredtent.net

ww.redtentdirectory.com

www.deannalam.com

www.pinterest.com/dreamingaloudnt/in-the-red-tent

Facebook community pages

The Happy Womb

Red Tent Movement

Red tents Moon lodges Red tent temples

Women's Red Tents and Temples Worldwide

Things We Don't Talk About: The Red Tent Movie

Red Tents in Every Neighbourhood

The Moon Woman

Occupy Menstruation

Journey of Young Women

Red tent videos online

Lucy H. Pearce talking about red tents as part of DeAnna L'Am's Red Tent Summit 2014:
https://youtu.be/0ox5v5j8DXM

Lucy H. Pearce talking about empowering girls as part of DeAnna L'Am's Empowering Girls Summit 2015:
https://youtu.be/esT6KJc-w9w

Introduction to red tents and celebrating menarche:
http://youtube/1enWN7n8l3E

DeAnna L'am's Red Tent in California:
http://www.youtube.com/watch?v=CQ39pZC6DRs

http://wn.com/The_Red_Tent

Books

Moon time

Red Moon: Understanding and using the creative sexual and spiritual gifts of the menstrual cycle—Miranda Gray

The Optimized Woman—Miranda Gray

The Woman's Quest—Unfolding Women's Path of Power and Wisdom—Alexandra Pope (from www.wildgenie.com)

The Wild Genie: The Healing Power of Menstruation—Alexandra Pope

Thirteen Moons—Rachael Hertogs

The Wise Wound—Penelope Shuttle & Peter Redgrove

Alchemy for Women—Penelope Shuttle & Peter Redgrove

Cycle to the Moon: celebrating the menstrual trinity—Veronika Sophia Robinson

Code Red: know your flow, unlock your superpowers + create a bloody amazing life. Period—Lisa Lister

Grandmother Moon: Lunar Magic In Our Lives—Spells, Rituals, Goddesses, Legends and Emotions—Z. Budapest

Her Blood is Gold: Celebrating the Power of Menstruation—Lara Owen

Songs of Bleeding—Spider

Menarche

Reaching for the Moon: a girl's guide to her female cycles (a soulful guide for girls aged 9–14)—Lucy H. Pearce

Menarche: A Journey into Womanhood—Rachael Hertogs

Mother-Daughter Wisdom: Understanding the Crucial Links Between Mothers, Daughters and Health—Dr Christiane Northrup

Celebrating Girls—Virginia Beane-Rutter

A Blessing not a Curse: A mother daughter guide to the transition from child to woman—Jane Bennett

A Diva's Guide to Getting Your First Period—DeAnna L'am with gloriously creative and bright illustrations by Jessica Jarman-Hayes

The Thundering Years: Rituals and Sacred Wisdom for Teens—Julie Tallard Johnson

Raising Girls— Steve Biddulph

The Seven Sacred Rites of Menarche—Kristi Meisenbach Boylan

Becoming Peers—DeAnna L'am

Becoming a Woman: A Guide for Girls Approaching Menstruation—Jane Hardwicke Collings

Circle Round: Raising Children in Goddess Traditions—Starhawk, Diane Baker, Anne Hill, Sara Ceres Boore

A Time To Celebrate: A Celebration of a Girl's First Menstrual Period—Joan Morais

For the text of a whole menarche book online:
www.moonandearthconnections.com/menstruationbooklets.htm

www.journeyofyoungwomen.org

www.deannalam.com

www.pinterest.com/dreamingaloudnt/empowering-girls

Menopause and croning

The Wisdom of Menopause—Dr Christiane Northrup

Red Moon Passage—Bonnie Horrigan

The Change—Germaine Greer

Crone—Barbara Walker

Passage To Power: Natural Menopause Revolution—Leslie Kenton

Crones Don't Whine: Concentrated Wisdom for Juicy Women—Jean Shinoda Bolen

New Menopausal Years: The Wise Woman Way—*Alternative Approaches for Women 30–90*—Susun Weed

Natural Solutions to Menopause: How to stay healthy before, during and beyond the menopause—Marilyn Glenville

Goddesses Never Age: The Secret Prescription for Radiance, Vitality and Wellbeing—Dr Christiane Northrup

www.daisynetwork.org.uk

Sacred Menopause—Facebook Group

Miscarriage and stillbirth

uk-sands.org

Still Standing Magazine

www.talkbirth.com

Footprints on My Heart: a memoir of miscarriage and pregnancy after loss—Molly Remer

Ritual, ceremony and celebration

www.ritualwell.org—for Jewish based rituals

www.paganwiccan.about.com—for Pagan and Earth based ceremonies

www.blessingwaybook.com

www.pinterest.com/dreamingaloudnt/the-happy-womb

www.pinterest.com/dreamingaloudnt/blessingway

Birthrites—Jackie Singer

For rites of passage ceremony for every part of the fertility journey.

Moon Rites—ritual, myth and magic for the modern moon goddess—Spiraldancer

Mother Rising: the Blessingway Journey into Motherhood—Cortlund, Lucke & Watelet

Mother Blessings: Honoring Women Becoming Mothers—Anna Stewart

Blessingways: A Guide to Mother-Centered Baby Showers—Shari Maser

The Blessingway: creating a beautiful blessingway ceremony—Veronika Sophia Robinson

Body love and sex

Doodle your down there—a colouring book of genitals!

Cunt Loving Quest e-course—www.cherishthecunt.com

Woman is a River e-course—www.pixiecampbell.com

Read my Lips: A Complete Guide to the Vagina and Vulva—Debbie Herbenick & Vanessa Schick

Wild Feminine—Tami Lynn Kent

Cunt—Inga de Muscio

Vagina: a new biography—Naomi Wolf

The Vagina Monologues—Eve Ensler

Bodies—Susie Orbach

Women who Love Sex—Gina Ogden

Women's Anatomy of Arousal—Sherri Winston

The Hite Report—Shere Hite

The Sexual Practices of the Quodoshka—Amara Charles

Women's herbals

Herbal Healing for Women—Rosemary Gladstar

Neal's Yard Natural Remedies—Susan Curtis

Holistic Women's Herbal—K Campion

Wise Woman's Herbal for the Childbearing Year—Susun Weed

Letting in the Wild Edges—Glennie Kindred

Women's bodies, womb health and healing

The Uterine Health Companion—Dr. Eve Agee

Natural Solutions to PCOS: How to eliminate your symptoms and boost your fertility—Marilyn Glenville

Period Repair Manual: Natural Treatment for Better Hormones and Better Periods—Lara Briden

Women's Bodies, Women's Wisdom—Dr Christiane Northrup

Woman's Health in Woman's Hands—D. Cooper

The Hormone Cure—Dr Sara Gottfried

Yoni Shakti: a woman's guide to power and freedom through yoga and tantra—Uma Dinsmore Tuli

Hands on Health—Paula Youmell

You Can Heal Your Life—Louise. L. Hay

Woman Heal Thyself: an ancient healing system for contemporary women—Jeanne Elizabeth Blumm

www.womentowomen.com

Contraception and fertility

The Pill: Are you sure it's for you?—Jane Bennett and Alexandra Pope

The Birth of the Pill: How Four Pioneers Reinvented Sex and Launched a Revolution—Jonathan Eig

Sweetening the Pill: or How We Got Hooked on Hormonal Birth Control—Holly Griggs Spall

Taking Charge of your Fertility—Toni Weschler

Conscious Conception—Jeannine Parvati Baker

Women's wisdom—nourishing books that honour the feminine

The Rainbow Way: cultivating creativity in the midst of motherhood—Lucy H. Pearce

Moods of Motherhood: the inner journey of mothering—Lucy H. Pearce

Succulent Wild Woman: dancing with your wonder-full self—SARK

The Woman's Comfort Book—Jennifer Louden

The Woman's Retreat Book—Jennifer Louden

Shakti Woman: Feeling Our Fire, Healing Our World—*The New Female Shamanism*—Vicki Noble

Embodying the Feminine—Chameli Ardagh

Body of Wisdom—Hilary Hart

Maps to Ecstasy: The Healing Power of Movement—Gabrielle Roth

Circle of Stones—Judith Duerk

Women Who Run with the Wolves—Clarissa Pinkola Estes

Untie the Strong Woman—Clarissa Pinkola Estes

Ix Chel Wisdom—Shonagh Home

Keys to the Open Gate: A Woman's Spirituality Sourcebook—Kimberley Snow

Womanrunes—Molly Remer

She Walks in Beauty—*A Woman's Journey Through Poems*—selected by Caroline Kennedy

Journey to the Dark Goddess—Jane Meredith

Kissing the Hag: the dark goddess and the unacceptable nature of women

Jaguar Woman—Lynn V. Andrews

The Heart of the Labyrinth—Nicole Schwab

Red Hot and Holy—Sera Beak

The Woman in the Body—Emily Martin

Herstory—Free e-book of women's history available from www.moonsong.com.au

INDEX

ABOUT THE AUTHOR

LUCY H. PEARCE is the author of numerous life-changing non-fiction books for women, including: *Full Circle Health: integrated health charting for women*; *Burning Woman*; *The Rainbow Way: cultivating creativity in the midst of motherhood* and *Moon Time: harness the ever-changing energy of your menstrual cycle*. 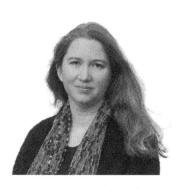 Her girls' book, *Reaching for the Moon: a girl's guide to her cycles* is now also available in French, Spanish, Polish and Dutch.

Lucy's work is dedicated to supporting women's empowered, embodied expression through her writing, teaching and art. She lives in East Cork, Ireland, where she runs Womancraft Publishing – creating life-changing, paradigm-shifting books by women, for women.

www.lucyhpearce.com

WOMANCRAFT PUBLISHING

Life-changing, paradigm-shifting books
by women, for women.

WWW.WOMANCRAFTPUBLISHING.COM

Sign up to the mailing list for discounts and see samples of
forthcoming titles before anyone else.

(f) WomancraftPublishing

(y) WomancraftBooks

(o) Womancraft_Publishing

If you have enjoyed this book, please leave a review
at your favourite retailer or Goodreads.

Also from Womancraft

Full Circle Health: integrated health charting for women

by Lucy H. Pearce

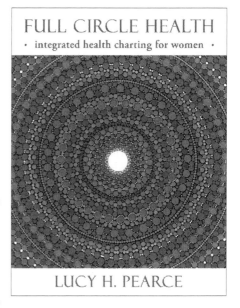

Welcome to *Full Circle Health*. A creative approach to holistic health for all who love planners, trackers and bullet journals to guide and support you in a greater understanding of your physical, mental and emotional health.

Whether menstruating or not, pregnant or post-partum, *Full Circle Health* provides a highly flexible, deeply supportive way of tracking your health, whatever your current health conditions.

Find guidance on:

- Cycles and why they are important for women's health
- Health charting a variety of physical and mental health conditions
- Menstrual charting
- Lunar charting
- Dream charting
- Guided journaling

With 35 daily charting spreads, a monthly habit tracker, planner, and charting grid, this integrated tool will help you to track symptoms, medication, self-care, energy levels, build positive health habits and mindful awareness.

Burning Woman

by Lucy H. Pearce

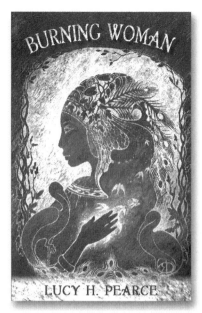

A breath-taking and controversial woman's journey through history — personal and cultural — on a quest to find and free her own power.

Uncompromising and all-encompassing, Pearce uncovers the archetype of the Burning Women of days gone by — Joan of Arc and the witch trials, through to the way women are burned today in cyber bullying, acid attacks, shaming and burnout, fearlessly examining the roots of Feminine power —what it is, how it has been controlled, and why it needs to be unleashed on the world during our modern Burning Times.

With contributions from leading burning women of our era: Isabel Abbott, ALisa Starkweather, Shiloh Sophia McCloud, Molly Remer, Julie Daley, Bethany Webster . . .

A must-read for all women! A life-changing book that fills the reader with a burning passion and desire for change.

Glennie Kindred, author of *Earth Wisdom*

Moon Dreams Diary

by Starr Meneely

Nurturing mindfulness, reflectiveness and awareness of our body, feelings, menstrual cycle, and the cycle of the moon, *Moon Dreams* is a simple yet powerful tool in the form of a beautifully illustrated week-on-two-page diary.

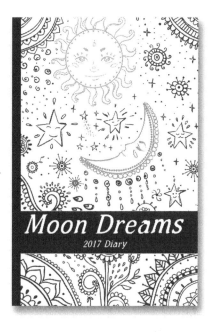

- O 52-week diary
- O Space to doodle
- O Beautiful illustrations to colour
- O Information on charting your cycle
- O Learn about the moon's phases and how they affect you
- O Quotations to inspire and uplift
- O Private space to reflect

This journal will set young women on a path of mindfulness, self-love and connection with the wild, beautiful, natural world around them. Moon Dreams has the potential to be life changing; it reclaims our menstrual cycle as a sacred, powerful experience, rather than the revolting weakness that modern society seems to view it as. Every woman needs to get her hands on a Moon Dreams journal!

Lucy AitkenRead, *Lulastic and the Hippyshake*

Reaching for the Moon: a girl's guide to her cycles

by Lucy H. Pearce

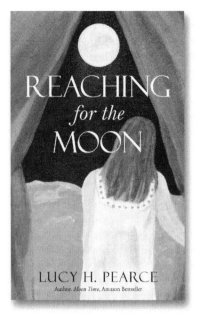

The girls' version of Lucy H. Pearce's Amazon bestselling book *Moon Time*. For girls aged 9-14, as they anticipate and experience their body's changes. *Reaching for the Moon* is a nurturing celebration of a girl's transformation to womanhood.

Beginning with an imaginary journey into the red tent, a traditional place of women's wisdom, gifts and secrets of womanhood are imparted in a gentle lyrical way. along with practical advice.

Now also available in the following translations:

Reiken naar de Maan (Dutch)
Rejoindre la Lune (French)
W Rytmie Księżyca (Polish)

A message of wonder, empowerment, magic and beauty in the shared secrets of our femininity . . . written to encourage girls to embrace their transition to womanhood in a knowledgeable, supported, loving way.

thelovingparent.com

The Other Side of the River: stories of women, water and the world,

by Eila Kundrie Carrico

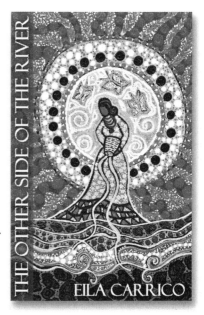

A deep searching into the ways we become dammed and how we recover fluidity. It is a journey through memory and time, personal and shared landscapes to discover the source, the flow and the deltas of women and water.

Rooted in rivers, inspired by wetlands, sources and tributaries, this book weaves its path between the banks of memory and story, from Florida to Kyoto, storm-ravaged New Orleans to London, via San Francisco and Ghana. We navigate through flood and drought to confront the place of wildness in the age of technology.

Part memoir, part manifesto, part travelogue and part love letter to myth and ecology, *The Other Side of the River* is an intricately woven tale of finding your flow . . . and your roots.

An instant classic for the new paradigm.

Lucia Chiavola Birnbaum, award-winning author and Professor Emeritus

The Heroines Club: a mother-daughter empowerment circle,

by Melia Keeton-Digby

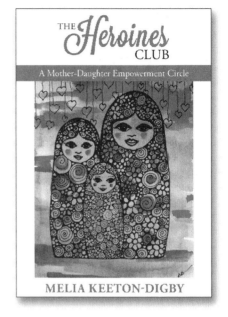

Nourishing guidance and a creative approach for mothers and daughters, aged 7+, to learn and grow together through the study of women's history. Each month focuses on a different heroine, featuring athletes, inventors, artists, and revolutionaries from around the world— including Frida Kahlo, Rosalind Franklin, Amelia Earhart, Anne Frank, Maya Angelou and Malala Yousafzai as strong role models for young girls to learn about, look up to, and be inspired by.

The Heroines Club is truly a must-have book for mothers who wish to foster a deeper connection with their daughters. As mothers, we are our daughter's first teacher, role model, and wise counsel. This book should be in every woman's hands, and passed down from generation to generation.
Wendy Cook, founder and facilitator of Mighty Girl Art

Liberating Motherhood: birthing the purplestockings movement

by Vanessa Olorenshaw

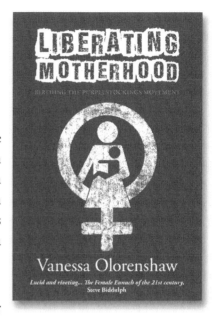

If it is true that there have been waves of feminism, then mothers' rights are the flotsam left behind on the ocean surface of patriarchy. Mothers are in bondage – and not in a 50 Shades way.

Liberating Motherhood discusses our bodies, our minds, our labour and our hearts, exploring issues from birth and breastfeeding to mental health, economics, politics, basic incomes and love and in doing so, broaches a conversation we've been avoiding for years: how do we value motherhood?

Highly acclaimed by leading parenting authors, academics and activists, with a foreword by Naomi Stadlen, founder of Mothers Talking and author of *What Mothers Do*, and *How Mothers Love*.

Lucid and riveting... This is The Female Eunuch of the 21st century.
Steve Biddulph, bestselling author of *Raising Boys, Raising Girls*, and *The Secret of Happy Children*

Liberating Motherhood is an important contribution to a vital debate of our times. Vanessa Olorenshaw speaks with warmth, wit and clarity, representing lives and voices unheard for too long.
Shami Chakrabarti, author of *On Liberty*, former director of Liberty and formerly 'the most dangerous woman in Britain'

The Heart of the Labyrinth

by Nicole Schwab

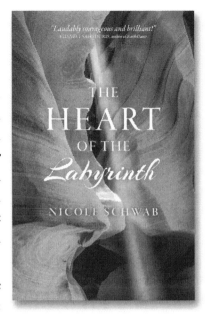

Reminiscent of Paulo Coelho's masterpiece *The Alchemist* and Lynn V. Andrew's acclaimed *Medicine Woman* series, *The Heart of the Labyrinth* is a beautifully evocative spiritual parable, filled with exotic landscapes and transformational soul lessons.

As everything she thought she knew about herself disintegrates: her health, career, family and identity, Maya embarks on a journey of discovery to the land of her ancestors. Coming face-to-face with her subconscious belief that being a woman is a threat, she understands that to step into wholeness she will have to reclaim the sacred feminine fire burning in her soul.

Once in a while, a book comes along that kindles the fire of our inner wisdom so profoundly, the words seem to leap off the page and go straight into our heart. If you read only one book this year, this is it.

Dean Ornish, M.D, President, Preventive Medicine Research Institute, Author of *The Spectrum*

Moods of Motherhood: the inner journey of mothering,

by Lucy H. Pearce

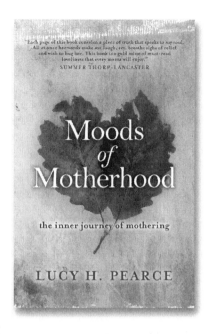

Moods of Motherhood charts the inner journey of motherhood, giving voice to the often nebulous, unspoken tumble of emotions that motherhood evokes: tenderness, frustration, joy, grief, anger, depression and love. Lucy H. Pearce explores the taboo subjects of maternal ambiguity, competitiveness, and the quest for perfection, offering support, acceptance, and hope to mothers everywhere. Though the story is hers, it could be yours.

This fully-updated second edition features 23 new pieces including posts written for her popular blog, Dreaming Aloud, her best-loved magazine columns and articles, and many other original pieces. This is a book full of Lucy's trademark searing honesty and raw emotions, which have brought a global following of mothers to her work.

Lucy's frank and forthright style paired with beautiful, haunting language and her talent for storytelling will have any parent nodding, crying and laughing along – appreciating the good and the bad, the hard and the soft, the light and the dark. A must-read for any new parent.

Zoe Foster, JUNO magazine

Dirty & Divine: a transformative journey through tarot

by Alice B. Grist

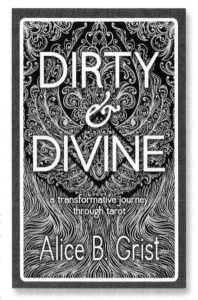

There is something sacred within you, in all that you are and all that you do. In a mix of you that is everyday dirty, and spiritually divine, there is something so perfect, something more. Welcome to your journey back home; to your dirty, divine passage back to you.

Wherever you are, whether beginner or seasoned tarot practitioner, *Dirty & Divine* is written for you, to accompany you on a powerful personal intuitive journey to plumb the depths of your existence and encompass the spectrum of wisdom that the cards can offer.

Dirty & Divine is a tarot-led vision quest to reclaiming your femininity in all its lucid and colourful depths.

Alice has been my go-to woman for tarot readings for years now, because her truth, knowledge + wisdom are the REAL DEAL.
Lisa Lister, author of *Love your Lady Landscape*

The Goddess in You

by Patrícia Lemos and Ana Afonso

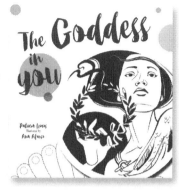

The Goddess in You is especially created for girls aged 9-14 years, offering a unique, interactive approach to establishing cycle awareness, positive health and well-being. It contains thirteen beautifully designed cycle mandalas, each illustrated with a goddess from Greek mythology.

Easy to understand and attractive to use, this powerful book celebrates what it means to be a girl growing into womanhood.

- 13 double-sided cycle mandalas illustrated with goddesses

- Instructions for use

- An introduction to the 13 featured Greek goddesses

- A basic, age-appropriate introduction to the menstrual cycle

- Self-care tips for health and well-being

A beautiful resource... Both psychologically sophisticated and delightfully simple to use, I warmly recommend this book to girls, parents and schools.
Jane Bennett, author of *A Blessing Not a Curse*

A simple and beautiful invitation to help girls build a relationship with their menstrual cycle. We highly recommend this book for all young menstruating women.
Alexandra Pope and Sjanie Hugo Wurlitzer, co-authors of *Wild Power*

Printed in Great Britain
by Amazon